DRUGS FOR THE GUT

A Practical Guide to Gastrointestinal and Liver Therapy

DRUGS FOR THE GUT

A Practical Guide to Gastrointestinal and Liver Therapy

Peter Prichard, Robert Walt and Roger Chapman

WB SAUNDERS COMPANY LIMITED
London Philadelphia Toronto Sydney Tokyo

WB Saunders Company Ltd
24–28 Oval Road, London NW1 7DX, UK

WB Saunders Company
The Curtis Center, Independence Square West
Philadelphia, PA 19106–3399, USA

Harcourt Brace & Company, 55 Horner Avenue
Toronto, Ontario M8Z 4X6, Canada

Harcourt Brace & Company, Australia
30–52 Smidmore Street, Marrickville, NSW 2204, Australia

Harcourt Brace & Company, Japan
Ichibancho Central Building, 22-1
Ichibancho, Chiyoda-ku, Tokyo, 102, Japan

A CIP record for this book is available from the British Library

ISBN 0–7020–1802–3

Typeset in Palatino by Laserscript, Mitcham, Surrey
Printed in Great Britain by WBC, Bridgeend, Mid Glamorgan

CONTENTS

1.4 Small and Large Intestine

PREFACE

Drugs with proven efficacy are relatively new to gastroenterology. It is difficult to keep up with the development of new agents, and new indications for older drugs. When twenty years ago there was little specific treatment for liver disease who would have predicted the agents now used in viral hepatitis, primary biliary cirrhosis and bleeding varices. The development of specific anti-ulcer drugs has mushroomed to produce numerous agents used in the control of upper gastrointestinal disease. The alternative therapies in inflammatory bowel disease have multiplied and the use of nutritional support has justifiably found an important place in the therapy of gastrointestinal and other chronic illness. Generalists can not be expected to remember all the names, doses and indications and the latter change rapidly. The role of *Helicobacter pylori* treatment changes so fast that few can have more than a superficial understanding. This small manual should help generalists and trainee gastroenterologists in managing common and rare gastrointestinal problems. The emphasis is on drug therapy but in many instances drugs are unhelpful while other physical or endoscopic interventions could be effective. This is not a textbook of gastrointestinal disease but in some instances therapeutic activity can only be understood if some of the pathogenesis of disease is known. Hence in the first section we have striven to balance disease descriptions and investigation with details on the commonly used drugs including practical tips which come from frequent use. Where common GI therapies are mentioned the basic pharmacological data including doses are given in the second edition of the book. In a few instances we recommend treatments which may not be licensed (in one country of another) for particular indications, but it is experience of treating patients as well as clinical trial evidence which we hope to impart. All doses must be checked. Even very careful proof reading sometimes allows glaring misprints.

NOTICE

SECTION A

Oesophagus

1.1

1.1.1

Oesophageal Reflux Disease

EPIDEMIOLOGY AND PATHOLOGY

Oesophageal reflux is uncommon in the Far East yet appears to be becoming more common in the West, either through better or more frequent recognition or because the disease itself is more common. It is symptomatic in up to 40% of the general population whether or not they are attending a doctor. Symptoms are closely, although not always directly, related to reflux of acidic gastric contents and therapy has primarily been aimed at reduction of acid secretion. Acid secretion is not abnormal in most patients with reflux symptoms. Alkaline reflux can occur after gastric surgery and possibly in the intact stomach and therapeutic measures here are less effective. The underlying problem in gastrooesophageal reflux is a lax lower oesophageal sphincter. Patients with severe reflux symptoms and oesophagitis have lower sphincter pressures than others, thus allowing gastric contents to reflux. Spontaneous relaxations of the sphincter are more common in reflux disease. In many cases a more generalized defect in oesophageal motility disturbs the natural ability of the oesophagus to clear the refluxate, increasing the amount of time acid contents lie in the oesophagus. Hiatus hernia is associated but is not the primary problem (see *1.1.3 Hiatus Hernia*).

Notes

PRESENTATION

Heartburn is the major symptom, but epigastric pain after meals is also common. Symptoms provoked by bending or lying down, by fatty or rich meals, and by alcohol are frequent. Waterbrash is not uncommon and occasionally chest pain indistinguishable from cardiac pain may present. Recent weight gain is a common feature and heartburn occurs in pregnancy. Substantial regurgitation can occur and nocturnal reflux is believed to produce "asthma" or episodic nocturnal breathlessness in some.

If oesophagitis is severe, patients may present with haematemesis, anaemia and even dysphagia if a stricture has developed. In some patients dysphagia is a symptom of reflux without physical obstruction.

INVESTIGATIONS

Careful history taking and possibly therapeutic trials are the major diagnostic procedures. No single investigation is adequate or practical for most patients. Endoscopy which demonstrates strictures, gross oesophagitis and hiatus hernia (see *1.1.3*) can be normal in patients with heartburn due to reflux. pH monitoring over 24 hours identifies patients with non-specific symptoms associated with acid reflux and offers an opportunity for patients to indicate symptoms on the recording device. It may miss patients in whom tolerance to reflux is poor and it does not identify alkaline refluxers. Studies with radiolabelled meals can also demonstrate reflux, but are rarely used. Manometry is useful to identify motility

Notes

disorders, but treatments for the latter are unsatisfactory and it is debatable whether manometry should be considered outside specialist units. Barium meal frequently demonstrates reflux even in patients without symptoms. Symptomatic trials with *omeprazole 40–80 mg daily for 5 days* have been recommended and can identify patients whose symptoms respond to acid reduction. Routine investigation is recommended before surgery (to ensure that the patients referred have genuine reflux) and where alternative important diagnoses (ulcer or cancer) are suspected. Endoscopy is important in patients with dysphagia for therapy as well as diagnosis. Some argue that endoscopy should be routine so as to identify patients with Barrett's oesophagus (see *1.1.2*).

MANAGEMENT

Symptomatic therapy is the mainstay and will remain so until it has been conclusively demonstrated that treatment of oesophagitis prevents the development of complications. *Antacids* and *alginates* are commonly used with apparently good response. Such agents are available without prescription and many patients have already tried these remedies before seeking further help. The next stage in management is to decrease acid secretion and it is clear that the most potent antisecretory agents *proton pump inhibitors omeprazole, lansoprazole,* and *pantoprazole* produce better symptomatic responses than the *H_2-receptor antagonists cimetidine, ranitidine, famotidine, nizatidine,* and *roxatidine.* These drugs are used in the recommended doses for peptic ulcer, but nocturnal

Notes

dosing is not logical in this condition where reflux occurs mostly during the day. Treatment is also used to heal oesophagitis, and again the proton pump inhibitors work best. High-dose H_2-receptor antagonist therapy, for example 300 mg ranitidine four times daily, may be equally effective but the simplicity and efficacy of omeprazole 20 mg or lansoprazole 30 mg daily makes them first-line therapy. In some patients 40 mg omeprazole is required. In many patients symptoms rapidly recur on stopping the antisecretory treatment and in some long-term therapy is required. Studies of oesophagitis have shown that proton pump inhibitors are reasonably successful at reducing relapse rates, whereas H_2-receptor antagonists are much less effective. It appears that 10 mg omeprazole or 15 mg lansoprazole daily long-term is effective at preventing recurrent oesophageal reflux disease. The prokinetic agent *cisapride* has also been shown to help here, but direct comparisons against proton pump blockers have not been performed. *Cisapride 5–10 mg three times daily* is about as effective as the H_2-receptor antagonists in controlling symptoms and encouraging healing of oesophagitis and thus can be assumed to be less effective than proton pump inhibitors. It should be considered in patients who for some reason can not take antisecretory treatment, and in some cases may be a useful adjunct.

Dysphagia due to oesophageal stricture is generally treated endoscopically by dilatation, and in many patients multiple dilatations are required. Omeprazole 20 mg daily has been shown to reduce the requirement for repeated dilatation of oesophageal strictures, and no other drug has yet been shown to achieve this.

Notes

Oesophageal ulcers are treated as above for reflux oesophagitis but fear of malignancy masquerading as a benign lesion means that repeat endoscopy and biopsy is required after 2 months of treatment (see *1.2.4 Gastric Ulcer*).

1.1.2

Barrett's Oesophagus

Barrett's oesophagus is diagnosed when the normal squamous mucosa of the oesophagus is replaced by columnar mucosa.

EPIDEMIOLOGY AND PATHOLOGY

The normal squamous mucosa undergoes columnar transformation and looks more like gastric-fundal mucosa, hence the common term of gastric-lined oesophagus. The belief is that long-standing reflux of gastric contents leads to this change and that patients with Barrett's are at the severe end of the reflux spectrum. However, it is clear from endoscopic studies that between 4 and 10% of the population have Barrett's oesophagus of some extent. The mucosal abnormality almost always starts at the usual gastrooesophageal mucosal junction and may extend up the oesophagus in a confluent tube or in tongues or small islands. The extent is usually measured as distance above the gastrooesophageal junction and this measure is used to demonstrate whether a treatment has any effect on the disease. There is a problem ensuring that all endoscopists

Notes

agree on the site of the gastrooesophageal junction, which is further complicated if hiatus hernia is present. Thus most people will diagnose Barrett's oesophagus only when at least 3 cm of oesophagus is involved, and many insist on 5 cm. The importance of the diagnosis is that there is an increased risk of oesophageal adenocarcinoma in such patients. The risk of developing adenocarcinoma of 1 in 50 years' follow-up is probably proportional to the extent of Barrett's mucosa, but this is disputed.

PRESENTATION

Patients with Barrett's oesophagus are usually indistinguishable from the typical dyspeptics attending for endoscopy. Thus the diagnosis may be made incidentally or in association with oesophagitis.

INVESTIGATIONS

The diagnosis is usually clear at endoscopy unless severe oesophagitis obscures it. Histologic confirmation of columnar mucosa in biopsies taken from the oesophagus is necessary for absolute diagnosis. Barium radiology, pH measurements and manometry are not able to make this diagnosis.

MANAGEMENT

There is no consensus on how Barrett's should be managed. There is certainly no treatment that has been shown to categorically reverse the mucosal changes or reduce the risk of adenocarcinoma. Some argue that once

Notes

a diagnosis has been made patients should be kept under endoscopic surveillance with multiple biopsies being taken to identify dysplastic change. While this procedure can identify the development of adenocarcinoma, it has not been shown to improve outlook overall, and from a population basis can not be generally recommended. *Omeprazole 20–40 mg* daily for years has been reported to be associated with the development of squamous mucosal islands within the Barrett's mucosa. *Lansoprazole* or *pantoprazole* would be expected to produce similar change. The length of the Barrett's segment, however, is probably not significantly reduced by such therapy. The data so far are preliminary and based on relatively small numbers of patients but are reasonably consistent. The development of squamous islands, however, may simply be a cosmetic change and may not be associated with a reduction in risk of adenocarcinoma. On the basis of present information, no medical treatment can be recommended specifically for Barrett's oesophagus. In patients with symptoms of reflux, treatment should be directed at the reflux (see *1.1.1 Oesophageal Reflux Disease*).

1.1.3

Hiatus Hernia

Hiatus hernia is diagnosed when part of the stomach protrudes above the diaphragm. A sliding hernia rides up through the hiatal orifice and the esophagogastric junction moves up with it. A paraoesophageal hernia signifies the protrusion of a part of the stomach alongside

Notes

the usual gastrooesophageal junction. Combinations occur but paraoesophageal herniation is relatively rare.

PRESENTATION

Paraoesophageal hernia can present with mechanical obstruction or intermittent volvulus leading to dysphagia and retrosternal discomfort. Fortunately the common hiatus hernia probably produces no symptoms *per se* but is associated with gastrooesophageal reflux and heartburn.

INVESTIGATIONS

Large paraoesophageal hernias may be found coincidentally on routine chest radiography when a fluid level is seen in a widened lower mediastinum. Sliding hernia is commonly diagnosed during endoscopy or at barium meal when it is often blamed (unfairly) for the patient's symptoms.

MANAGEMENT

No specific treatment is required for sliding hiatus hernia. Treatment may be needed for the associated reflux symptoms and is discussed in the separate section. Surgical repair is an important consideration in those with mechanical problems for which pharmacologic treatment is inappropriate.

Notes

1.1

1.1.4

Oesophageal Motility Disorders

DEFINITION

These disorders are characterized by disturbed oesophageal peristalsis as measured by manometry. The disturbance can be failure of relaxation of the lower oesophageal sphincter (achalasia, Chagas' disease), failure of coordinated contraction (corkscrew oesophagus), or spasm of oesophageal muscles (diffuse oesophageal spasm, nutcracker oesophagus).

EPIDEMIOLOGY AND PATHOGENESIS

Achalasia is the best defined motility syndrome although its cause remains unknown. It is found in approximately 1 per 100 000 adults. There is loss of ganglion cells within the myenteric plexus and fewer vasoactive intestinal polypeptide (VIP) fibers are seen. Diffuse thickening of the oesophageal wall and dilatation occur with time. The manometric abnormalities are inadequate relaxation and hypertonicity of the lower oesophageal sphincter. The pathology underlying diffuse oesophageal spasm and nutcracker oesophagus, two other motility problems associated with increased pressure, are unknown. The manometric abnormality is a characteristic high-amplitude contraction which may also be prolonged. Firm manometric diagnosis is often difficult because these contractions can occur normally. Chagas' disease, caused by infection with *Trypanosoma cruzi*, is endemic in tropical South America but is seen only in visitors from

Notes

these countries elsewhere. It produces a dilated oesophagus due to myenteric failure. In systemic sclerosis (scleroderma), motor disorders of the oesophagus are common (50–80%). Lack of peristalsis and reduced or absent lower oesophageal sphincter tone is characteristic and distinguishes the problem from achalasia.

PRESENTATION

Dysphagia and weight loss are the most prominent symptoms of achalasia, whereas retrosternal chest pain is more commonly the presenting feature in diffuse oesophageal spasm and nutcracker oesophagus. Regurgitation and nocturnal cough are a frequent result of oesophageal dilatation and absent peristalsis. A combination of reflux symptoms and dysphagia is typical in scleroderma.

INVESTIGATIONS

Endoscopy is not a particularly useful diagnostic investigation in these cases. Barium radiology can often demonstrate disturbed peristalsis, particularly tertiary contractions which are characteristically uncoordinated and are not uncommon in elderly patients. The definition of these diseases requires that manometry is performed as a confirmatory test. An erect chest radiograph may show the widened mediastinum and fluid-filled dilated oesophagus, and the absence of the gastric air-bubble is another clue to the diagnosis of achalasia.

Notes

1.1

MANAGEMENT

Definitive treatment is aimed at improving oesophageal emptying and is achieved by endoscopic pneumatic dilatation or by surgical myotomy. Pharmacological therapies are relatively ineffective and are inadequate for the long-term management of the average patient. They are worth trying while awaiting definitive treatment. *Isosorbide dinitrate* reduces lower oesophageal sphincter pressure and can produce short-lived symptomatic improvement. Calcium channel antagonists have also been used, without dramatic success. Reflux symptoms associated with scleroderma are treated as for uncomplicated reflux oesophagitis, although responses are less satisfactory.

1.1.5

Oesophageal Carcinoma

The two most common oesophageal cancers are squamous cell carcinoma and adenocarcinoma.

EPIDEMIOLOGY AND PATHOLOGY

Squamous oesophageal cancer has a marked geographic variation in incidence. Extremely common in China and Iran, it is relatively uncommon in Europe. This suggests that environmental factors play an important part in causation. Alcohol, cigarette smoking, diet, genetic factors, and associated diseases all play some role. Barrett's oesophagus is associated with a higher incidence of

Notes

adenocarcinoma, whereas iron deficiency anaemia is associated with high squamous lesions. The two histologic types mentioned above seem to relate to different factors. Squamous carcinoma is not changing but adenocarcinoma is becoming more common. Squamous carcinoma is radiosensitive but adenocarcinoma responds poorly.

PRESENTATION

Dysphagia arises as the tumour spreads circumferentially restricting the oesophageal lumen. Solid food, often bread or meat, tends to stick first and occasionally patients can localize the level of the stricture. It is remarkable how small the oesophageal lumen can shrink to in some cases without severe symptoms. Eventually dysphagia for liquids with regurgitation occurs and weight loss is a prominent feature. Iron deficiency anaemia is not infrequent and pain can occur either on swallowing or through mediastinal involvement. Patients generally present late and spread to supraclavicular lymph nodes may be detectable.

INVESTIGATIONS

Endoscopy is the investigation of choice, although some recommend a barium swallow first in an attempt to avoid perforation of an unexpectedly high oesophageal stricture. Biopsies can be taken and therapeutic measures applied. When surgery is contemplated, computed tomography (CT), magnetic resonance imaging (MRI), or endoscopic oesophageal ultrasonography is advisable to determine which other mediastinal structures are

Notes

involved. The liver should be clear of metastases by ultrasonography if surgery is being considered.

MANAGEMENT

For most patients only palliative treatment is available. The options include endoscopic intubation, radiotherapy (for squamous lesions only), surgery, or endoscopic ablation therapy with either alcohol injection or laser. The choice depends on available skills rather than evidence that one therapy outshines another. Where curative surgery is feasible the outcomes are best. Prolonged remission can also be achieved with radiotherapy although eventual recurrence is likely. There are no pharmacologic interventions that can help, although some prescribe *steroids* for improved general well-being and others *proton pump inhibitors* to reduce reflux-induced pain.

1.1.6

Oesophageal Infections

Oesophagitis is generally secondary to reflux of acid but occasionally fungal infections (*Candida* mainly) and viruses (herpes simplex and cytomegalovirus) can invade oesophageal mucosa.

EPIDEMIOLOGY AND PATHOLOGY

Immunocompromised patients or those receiving oral or inhaled steroids commonly have oesophageal candidiasis,

Notes

whereas patients with human immunodeficiency virus (HIV) infection may have the other diseases. These oesophageal diseases are acquired immune deficiency syndrome (AIDS) defining diagnoses. *Candida* can frequently be identified on microscopy of smears and biopsies but has a characteristic clinical appearance of white plaques that bleed on washing at endoscopy. Cytomegalovirus can be identified by characteristic giant cells in the mucosa of the lower oesophagus and can occasionally produce ulcers which may be mistaken for oesophageal cancer. Herpes simplex usually produces fluid-filled vesicles, as are commonly seen in the mouth. The presence of *Candida* may obscure the macroscopic appearances of virus infection, so biopsies are recommended in all immunocompromised patients.

PRESENTATION

Pain on swallowing is the classic symptom, although pain may be present continuously. Difficulty swallowing is secondary to pain (odynophagia).

INVESTIGATIONS

Endoscopy is required for diagnosis and biopsies should be taken in all cases for viral culture and electron microscopy in addition to standard histology. The presence of obvious *Candida* should not prevent a search for other pathogens in patients with AIDS as multiple infections are common.

Notes

MANAGEMENT

Candidal oesophagitis is treated adequately with oral fluconazole, itraconazole, or ketoconazole but recurrence is frequent if the predisposing factor remains. In patients with severe immunodeficiency *Candida* may be difficult if not impossible to eradicate and amphotericin can be used systemically. Ganciclovir is frequently used for the viral infections, with limited success. Other newer antiviral drugs are in development and advice should be sought from an AIDS specialist. Symptomatic responses are adequate to monitor the success of treatment, although repeated endoscopy can be necessary if symptoms do not settle.

Stomach and Duodenum

1.2

1.2.1

Functional Dyspepsia

Functional dyspepsia defies present definition. It is also known as nonulcer dyspepsia. It is common and probably the cause of the majority of cases of uncomplicated dyspepsia. For the purposes of management it can be considered to include those symptoms which doctors believe are referrable to the upper gastrointestinal tract but where macroscopic endoscopic abnormalities are lacking. A large proportion of these patients have gastritis or duodenitis and approximately 50% or more are infected with *Helicobacter pylori*. Some patients have disturbed gastrointestinal motility with delayed gastric emptying or frequent tertiary contractions in the oesophagus. Identifying these associated features is not usually of diagnostic or therapeutic benefit.

EPIDEMIOLOGY AND PATHOLOGY

While there is no clear definition, the disease is difficult to study and little is known of its causes. Functional dyspepsia is likely to be a group of conditions, which presently can be roughly distinguished on symptomatology but not by cause:

1 Reflux like (where symptoms mimic gastrooesophageal reflux).
2 Dysmotility like (where belching, vomiting, early satiety, or fullness are predominant symptoms).
3 Ulcer like (where there is a relationship to food, and pain is sited in the epigastrium).

Notes

4 *H. pylori* associated (the role of the organism is unclear but there is an excess of infected individuals amongst sufferers of functional dyspepsia compared to the normal population).

PRESENTATION

Patients present with discomfort which may have the characteristic features outlined above. Psychologic factors should be explored because of the unsubstantiated belief that the disease may be predominantly psychosomatic.

INVESTIGATIONS

Endoscopy is required for formal diagnosis which depends on excluding mucosal disease. However, in practice, young patients with dyspepsia unassociated with *H. pylori* generally receive symptom-relieving treatment irrespective of diagnosis and in them the case for endoscopy is less clearcut. Many recommend that endoscopy should be performed only in young patients with serologic evidence of *H. pylori*.

MANAGEMENT

Treatment is difficult and aimed at symptom relief. If the patient falls into one of the relatively clearcut groups then treatment can be directed accordingly. Hence those with reflux symptoms should be treated in the first instance as for reflux oesophagitis (see *1.1.1 Oesophageal Reflux Disease*) and many will respond because in essence

Notes

they have reflux without oesophagitis. The dysmotility group can be started on a prokinetic agent such as *cisapride* which has been shown to be of some benefit in most studies. The ulcer-type group should be given anti-secretory treatment aiming to use the most cost-efficient therapy, which can range from *antacids* through *H_2-receptor antagonists* to *proton pump inhibitors*. There is much debate about whether to treat patients with *H. pylori* eradication therapy but at present there is no clear rationale for so doing and we do not recommend such treatment until evidence of benefit accumulates. Thus such patients should be treated symptomatically. Overall, symptom responses are generally incomplete and unsatisfactory irrespective of the type of symptom and many patients have successive therapeutic trials with all the agents mentioned above, and this proves unsuccessful in a large number. Satisfactory reassurance and support is probably of more therapeutic importance than drug treatment.

1.2.2

Delayed Gastric Emptying

Acute gastric dilatation is a rare association with other severe disease with concomitant metabolic disturbance. It is treated by dealing with the underlying condition and nasogastric suction. There is no pharmacologic therapy.

Delayed gastric emptying may follow vagotomy and is the reason a pyloroplasty is usually performed in conjunction with a truncal vagotomy. Metoclopramide (see *1.3.1 Vomiting*) and *cisapride* (see *2.1.5*) may be useful for symptomatic patients.

Notes

Diabetic gastroparesis is a rare motility disorder causing chronic gastric retention. Variable nausea, vomiting, fullness, and anorexia can be alleviated in some with drugs such as *cisapride*, metoclopramide, domperidone, or erythromycin.

1.2.3 Gastritis

Gastritis is a histologic finding, with an inflammatory infiltrate of lymphocytes, plasma cells, and polymorphs. Various classifications exist which help to predict etiology but may be of relatively little clinical value. Acute gastritis has a predominance of polymorphs and chronic gastritis a predominance of lymphocytes. Active chronic gastritis is almost always caused by *H. pylori* infection.

EPIDEMIOLOGY AND PATHOLOGY

Gastritis is common. Virtually all patients with peptic ulcers have associated gastritis and approximately 50% of those with dyspepsia have gastritis, often associated with *H. pylori*. The epidemiology of gastritis is poorly documented. Studies in Scandinavia have shown that it rarely disappears spontaneously and that it develops as patients age. Gastric cancer is believed to result from the evolution of active to atrophic gastritis with time. Atrophic gastritis is associated with loss of parietal cells and consequent decrease in acid secretion and intrinsic factor secretion. Autoimmune atrophic gastritis under-

Notes

pins the diagnosis of pernicious anaemia, where vitamin B_{12} malabsorption and achlorhydria are associated. It is not yet clear that treatment of gastritis has any virtue in either preventing symptoms or development of ulcer or cancer. Granulomatous gastritis is a rare association with Crohn's disease, tuberculosis, and histoplasmosis, and may be idiopathic. Eosinophilic gastritis where variably frequent eosinophils are found is usually of unknown etiology and is also uncommon.

PRESENTATION

Gastritis is diagnosed in patients undergoing endoscopy for any reason. It is therefore believed that the symptoms that provoke endoscopic investigation are caused by the gastritis, but this belief is without foundation. Many believe that it is an incidental finding of no symptomatic importance. Erosive gastritis associated with non-steroidal anti-inflammatory drug (NSAID) use may present with gastric bleeding, but its association with symptoms of dyspepsia in NSAID users is tenuous. Gastritis is a characteristic finding in the antrum in duodenal ulcer, associated in most cases with *H. pylori*. Gastritis is also present throughout the stomach in gastric ulcer and gastric cancer. Symptoms of these conditions are probably not referrable to the gastritis.

INVESTIGATIONS

If macroscopic erosive gastritis is seen at endoscopy the patient should be questioned about NSAID, aspirin, and alcohol use. *H. pylori*-associated gastritis is generally

Notes

invisible macroscopically and efforts to identify the organisms histologically or bacteriologically or by demonstrating urease activity (urea breath tests, biopsy urease tests) are required to make this diagnosis.

MANAGEMENT

Clinical benefit has not been demonstrated from treatment of gastritis and the authors do not recommend its treatment. NSAIDs should be stopped where possible. In general terms it is possible to only treat *H. pylori*-related gastritis and further study is required to tell whether this is worthwhile. For *H. pylori* eradication regimens see *2.1.8* (*Anti*-Helicobacter pylori *Treatment*). Granulomatous and eosinophilic gastritis have no specific treatments, although the former may respond to treatment of any identified cause.

1.2.4

GASTRIC ULCER

EPIDEMIOLOGY AND PATHOGENESIS

Gastric ulceration, a disease of young women at the end of the last century, has become a disease of the elderly. Ulcers are small breaks in the mucosa of the stomach, usually the lesser curve, and their cause is probably multifactorial. Acid plays a less important part in their pathogenesis and *H. pylori* is present in 70–85% of cases. NSAIDs are an important cause and account for approximately 30% of the complications of gastric ulcers.

Notes

The disease affects women more than men and women generally receive more NSAIDs than men at all ages. The epidemiological relationships with *H. pylori* are discussed under *Duodenal Ulcer* (see *1.2.5*).

PRESENTATION

Indigestion, dyspepsia, and epigastric pain are the common symptoms. The history is often inconsequential and a clinical diagnosis is probably impossible except by luck. Pain that is provoked by eating and that wakes the patient from sleep is a helpful pointer to the diagnosis. NSAIDs and aspirin probably account for up to 30% of gastric ulcers, so the drug history is important. Patients are more likely to be cigarette smokers and may have a family history of peptic ulcer. A small proportion of patients presents with one of three complications: haemorrhage, perforation, or pyloric stenosis. In about half of these cases there is no previous history of symptomatic ulcer disease. Physical signs, in the absence of complications, are negligible. Shock or postural hypotension with associated melena on rectal examination give good evidence of substantial haemorrhage. Board-like rigidity and other features of peritonism suggest perforation.

INVESTIGATION

Although barium radiology is an accurate diagnostic test for ulceration, endoscopy with biopsy is preferred. Gastric cancer can be indistinguishable macroscopically and therefore histology and cytology should be performed at

Notes

diagnosis and following treatment. In addition to biopsies of the ulcer, biopsies should be taken from the gastric antrum and body (especially if on acid suppression therapy) for urease test, histopathology, and possibly culture for *H. pylori*. Endoscopy is also superior to barium radiology in documenting other associated gastroduodenal pathology such as erosive gastritis.

Serum gastrin should be measured when Zollinger–Ellison syndrome is suspected. This rare syndrome is due to a gastrin-producing tumour (see *1.4.17 Secretory Diarrhoea*) and is associated with severe gastroduodenal ulceration that may be nonresponsive to standard acid suppression therapy.

MANAGEMENT

Clinical trials in gastric ulcer have shown that many drugs are effective compared with placebo. It should be possible to heal approximately 75% of all gastric ulcers in 8 weeks and upwards of 90% in 12 weeks using therapeutic doses of any of the groups of drugs considered below. When antisecretory therapy is used, healing rates are related more to the duration of therapy than to potency. Dietary manipulation and bedrest are no longer considered important but there is good reason to advise patients to stop smoking and to stop the use of NSAIDs and aspirin whenever possible. Endoscopic biopsies should be taken from the ulcer site after treatment, even when ulcers are healed.

Notes

Uncomplicated ulceration

Anti-*Helicobacter pylori* therapy

Treatment of gastric ulcers associated with *H. pylori* includes one or more antibiotics. These regimens may include one of the antisecretory agents plus one or more of amoxycillin, tetracycline, clarithromycin, and metronidazole. Bismuth compounds are also often included in such "eradication therapy". Gastric ulcers are much less likely to recur following such treatment. Successful eradication of *H. pylori* may even render a cure, provided NSAIDs were not being used at diagnosis and are not subsequently prescribed. The need for simple eradication regimens remains but existing ones have become first-line in *H. pylori*-positive gastric ulcer, unless NSAIDs are continued, in which case proton pump inhibitors are the most effective therapy. The advantages and disadvantages of eradication treatment are discussed in the section on duodenal ulcer (see *1.2.5*) and separately in *2.1.8* (*Anti-*Helicobacter pylori *Treatment*).

Reduce acidity

Traditional therapy aimed to buffer acid or limit its secretion. *Antacids* (see *2.1.1*) buffer secreted acid while they remain in the stomach and are frequently used for symptomatic relief. They can not be recommended as ulcer-healing therapy.

Anticholinergic agents inhibit acid secretion by blocking acetylcholine action on parietal cells at muscarinic receptors. They provide a minimal decrease in secretion and produce the expected unwanted effects of dry mouth, blurred vision, constipation, and urinary retention. They

Notes

are contraindicated in glaucoma. In an attempt to limit these unwanted effects selective antimuscarinic drugs were developed and *pirenzepine* (see *2.1.7*) has been marketed. This drug accelerates ulcer healing but standard anticholinergic side-effects occur at high dosage.

Histamine H_2-receptor antagonists revolutionized the treatment of ulcer in the mid-1970s. *Cimetidine 800 mg, ranitidine 300 mg, nizatidine 300 mg, famotidine 40 mg,* and *roxatidine 150 mg* are marketed examples (see *2.1.3 Histamine H_2-Receptor Antagonists*). They vary in potency and potential for drug interactions but in clinical terms they are equivalent. A course lasting 8 weeks is required for consistent gastric ulcer healing. The doses shown above are usually given in two divided doses, although single night-time use is probably equieffective.

Proton pump inhibitors prevent the exchange of hydrogen and potassium ions and powerfully decrease acid secretion. *Omeprazole 20 mg, lansoprazole 30 mg,* and *pantoprazole 40 mg* are currently available (see *2.1.4 Proton Pump Inhibitors*). There is little clinical difference between these agents. These drugs produce ulcer healing rates of about 70–80% after 4 weeks' therapy. Each is given in a single daily dose. Occasional patients require a higher dose, such as 40 mg omeprazole.

Mucosal protectives

A number of different agents fit into this category. Some like the *prostaglandin analogues* (*misoprostol 800 μg* (see *2.1.6*)) have mucosal effects as well as decreasing acid secretion, while with others the mechanisms of action are poorly understood. *Misoprostol* may be particularly effective in patients taking NSAIDs. Carbenoxolone was

Notes

the first nonantacid treatment and was popular in the early 1970s. Its mode of action is unclear but it has aldosterone-like effects which have limited its usefulness. Another compound derived from liquorice (Caved-S) was effective without mineralocorticoid activity. A few "non-absorbable" or poorly absorbed products are now available which accelerate ulcer healing. *Sucralphate* (see *2.1.10*) is a carbohydrate molecule with minimal buffering capacity but the ability to bind to exposed mucosal proteins, thus forming a scab and protecting from further damage. Bismuth was a relatively common constituent of antacids but fell into disrepute with the occurrence of significant encephalopathy after absorption. A few "non-absorbable" or poorly absorbed bismuth products are now available which accelerate ulcer healing. Ulcers also tend to relapse more slowly after healing, perhaps because bismuth interferes with *H. pylori*. Used as a single agent, however, bismuth drugs do not eradicate the organism (see *2.1.9 Colloidal Bismuth*).

Complicated ulceration

Perforation is an indication for emergency surgery. The defect should be repaired but no other surgical procedure should be necessary as medical therapy is so successful. Gastric ulcer excision may be difficult and gastrectomy is sometimes necessary. The management of haemorrhage from gastric ulcer is to maintain circulation. Patients are less tolerant of each successive period of hypotension. Many hospitals now use standard protocols as for duodenal ulcer (see *1.2.5*). Many endoscopists inject sclerosant adrenaline or alcohol, or apply diathermy

Notes

by some means, and such endoscopic intervention should limit the requirement for formal surgery in these protocols. However, the basic advice is that old people need early intervention while younger patients can tolerate more and longer periods of hypotension.

1.2.5

Duodenal Ulcer

EPIDEMIOLOGY AND PATHOGENESIS

Duodenal ulcers, rare in the late nineteenth century, had become commonplace by the mid-twentieth century. They are small breaks in the mucosa of the duodenum (usually the first part) and the cause is probably multifactorial. It is believed that they occur as a result of an imbalance between aggressive and protective elements acting in the duodenum. Acid was the traditional rogue and it is clear that patients with duodenal ulcer secrete more gastric acid than normal subjects. Acid activates pepsin which probably also plays a role in ulcerogenesis. The association with *H. pylori* (95%) has provoked a change in this perspective. One hypothesis now is that *H. pylori* infection of the gastric antrum results in hypergastrinaemia which in turn causes the acid hypersecretion. The ulcer in the duodenum develops only if an area of gastric metaplasia becomes infected with the organism resulting in erosive duodenitis. One of the factors leading to gastric metaplasia in the duodenum is believed to be gastric acid hypersecretion, thus it is possible to link duodenal ulcer and its multiple abnormalities through *H.*

Notes

pylori. Many aspects of the epidemiology of the disease can not be explained adequately on this hypothesis alone, so an open mind is recommended. The disease affects men more than women, although the prevalence of *H. pylori* is equal. The disease runs in families but few families harbour a particular type of organism. There are also patients with ulcers who have no evidence of *H. pylori* infection for whom another explanation is required. In many of these, NSAIDs play a part.

PRESENTATION

Indigestion, dyspepsia, or epigastric pain are common descriptions for the symptoms most commonly presenting. The history is often inconsequential and a clinical diagnosis is probably impossible except by luck. Pain relieved by eating or taking antacids, which wakes the patient from sleep and is not associated with bowel disturbance, is a helpful pointer to the diagnosis. Patients are more likely to be cigarette smokers and may have a family history of peptic ulcer. A small proportion of patients present with one of the three complications: haemorrhage, perforation, or pyloric stenosis. In about half of these cases there is no previous evidence of symptomatic ulcer disease. Physical signs, in the absence of complications, are negligible. Epigastric tenderness is common but unhelpful diagnostically. Shock or postural hypotension with associated melena on rectal examination give good evidence of substantial haemorrhage. Board-like rigidity and other features of peritonism suggest perforation, and a gastric splash some hours after eating is suggestive of pyloric outlet obstruction.

Notes

INVESTIGATION

Endoscopy or barium radiology remain the diagnostic tests. If endoscopy is undertaken, biopsies can be taken from the gastric antrum and body (especially if on acid suppression therapy) for urease test, histopathology, and possibly culture for *H. pylori*.

Serum gastrin should be measured when Zollinger–Ellison syndrome is suspected. This rare syndrome is due to a gastrin-producing tumour (see *1.4.17 Secretory Diarrhoea*) and is associated with severe gastroduodenal ulceration that may be nonresponsive to standard acid suppression therapy.

MANAGEMENT

Clinical trials in duodenal ulcer have demonstrated clearly that almost any drug is effective compared with placebo, despite vastly differing mechanisms of action. It should be possible to heal approximately 75% of all duodenal ulcers in 4 weeks and upwards of 90% in 8 weeks using therapeutic doses of any of the groups of drugs considered below. When antisecretory therapy is used healing rates are related to both the potency of the agent and the duration of therapy. Diet manipulation and bedrest are no longer considered important but there is ample scientific reason to advise patients to stop smoking and where possible to stop the use of NSAIDs and aspirin. These items of advice are additional to prescribing.

Notes

Uncomplicated ulceration

Anti-*Helicobacter pylori* therapy

Modern treatment of duodenal ulcers associated with *H. pylori* includes one or more antibiotics. These regimens may include one of the antisecretory agents plus two of either amoxycillin, clarithromycin, tetracycline and metronidazole. Bismuth compounds are also frequently included in such "eradication therapy". The main prompt for this change from traditional therapy has been the fact that duodenal ulcers are much less likely to recur following such treatment; indeed many believe that successful eradication of *H. pylori* renders a cure. The need for simple eradication regimens remains but existing ones have become first-line in duodenal ulcer. Combinations without metronidazole have the theoretical advantage of success when bacterial strains are resistant to nitroimidazoles. This may be particularly important in the developing world, where high levels of resistance are found. Reinfection in the West is unusual but may be a problem in countries where social overcrowding is the norm. Thus in such countries antimicrobial therapy may not offer such great advantages over conventional antisecretory therapy. In developed nations eradication therapy reduces the need for other therapies and prevents complications and hospitalization.

H. pylori treatments are discussed in *2.1.8* (*Anti-*Helicobacter pylori *Treatment*).

Reduce acidity

Traditional therapy aimed to buffer acid or limit its secretion. *Antacids* (see *2.1.1*) buffer secreted acid while

Notes

they remain in the stomach. Different formulations buffer more or less acid but no trials have demonstrated an advantage of one over another. Nevertheless a number of clinical trials have shown that regular antacid use accelerates duodenal ulcer healing. The disadvantage of antacids use is the frequency with which they are required, and many interfere with the absorption of other drugs. They are generally cheap, if inconvenient, and remain symptomatic therapy.

Anticholinergic agents inhibit acid secretion by blocking acetylcholine action on parietal cells at muscarinic receptors. They provide a minimal decrease in secretion and produce the expected unwanted effects of dry mouth, blurred vision, constipation, and urinary retention. They are contraindicated in glaucoma. In an attempt to limit these unwanted effects selective antimuscarinic drugs were developed and *pirenzepine* (see *2.1.7*) has been marketed. This drug accelerates ulcer healing but standard anticholinergic side-effects occur at high dosage.

Histamine H_2-receptor antagonists revolutionized the treatment of ulcer in the mid-1970s. They compete with histamine at receptors on parietal cells, decreasing acid secretion substantially. As they are competitive antagonists it is easiest to demonstrate their activity when competition is minimal (i.e. at night). Ulcer healing is accelerated even when the drugs are given as single doses at bedtime. It has been shown that the speed of healing is related to the extent of acid suppression and is hence dose related. *Cimetidine, ranitidine, nizatidine, famotidine,* and *roxatidine* are marketed examples (see *2.1.3 Histamine H_2-Receptor Antagonists*). They vary in

Notes

potency and potential for drug interactions but in clinical terms they are equivalent.

Proton pump inhibitors prevent the exchange of hydrogen and potassium ions and powerfully decrease acid secretion. *Omeprazole 20 mg, lansoprazole 30 mg,* and *pantoprazole 40 mg* are currently available (see *2.1.4 Proton Pump Inhibitors*). There is little clinical difference between these agents. These drugs produce ulcer healing rates of about 70–80% after 2 weeks of therapy.

Mucosal protectives

Many different agents fit into this category. Some, like the *prostaglandin analogues* (*misoprostol 800 μg* (see *2.1.6*)) have mucosal effects as well as decreasing acid secretion, while with others the mechanisms of action are poorly understood. Carbenoxolone was the first nonantacid treatment, popular in the early 1970s. Its mode of action is unclear but it has aldosterone-like effects which limit its usefulness. Another compound derived from liquorice (Caved-S) was effective without mineralocorticoid activity. *Sucralphate* (see *2.1.10*) is a carbohydrate molecule with minimal buffering capacity but the ability to bind to exposed mucosal proteins, thus forming a scab and protecting from further damage. Whether or not this is a more general effect through improved prostaglandin synthesis, sucralphate is able to heal duodenal ulcers. Bismuth was a relatively common constituent of antacids but fell into disrepute with the occurrence of significant encephalopathy after absorption. A few "nonabsorbable" or poorly absorbed products are now available which accelerate ulcer healing. Ulcers also tend to relapse more slowly after healing, perhaps because bismuth interferes

Notes

with *H. pylori*. Used as a single agent, however, bismuth drugs do not eradicate the organism (see *2.1.9 Colloidal Bismuth*).

Complicated ulceration

Perforation is an indication for emergency surgery. The defect should be repaired but no other surgical procedure should be necessary as medical therapy is so successful. In pyloric stenosis the requirement for intervention depends on symptoms. On occasion, patients settle with medical therapy which allows ulcer healing, a reduction in oedema, and hence a more patent pylorus. In other circumstances either endoscopic dilatation or surgical pyloroplasty is required. The management of haemorrhage from duodenal ulcer is more contentious. The most important aspect of this is speed of resuscitation and adequate maintenance of circulation. Patients tolerate each successive period of hypotension worse. Many hospitals now use standard protocols to aid management decisions based on evidence from clinical trials. Patients with significant bleeding should be admitted to hospital and some may argue that all patients should be admitted irrespective of severity as the risk of rebleeding is greatest in the first 24 hours. Many protocols then manage patients according to age above or below 60 years (see also *1.3.2.1 Upper Gastrointestinal Bleeding*). Those aged above 60 years receive intervention (surgery) after a single rebleed or when 4 units of blood or colloid over 24 hours have been required for volume replacement. Those aged under 60 years are allowed two rebleeds or 8 units of blood over 24

Notes

hours for volume replacement. Such a protocol has been shown to lead to low mortality rates in the elderly who are at greatest risk and to acceptably low intervention rates overall. Many endoscopists inject sclerosant adrenaline or alcohol, or apply diathermy by some means, and such endoscopic intervention should limit the requirement for formal surgery in these protocols. However, the basic advice of the protocol should be adhered to, namely that old people need early intervention whereas younger patients can tolerate more and longer periods of hypotension.

Common sense may push one towards withholding surgery from the oldest patients because they are so ill but data suggest that doing so worsens the outlook.

1.2.6 *Helicobacter pylori*

This organism is included here as a disease in its own right, although treatment is advised only in certain circumstances. The organism is associated with peptic ulcer, gastritis, duodenitis, ulcer-negative dyspepsia, gastric lymphoma, gastric carcinoma, short stature, and coronary artery disease. It is in the peptic ulcer group only that incontrovertible evidence demonstrates that treatment is worthwhile.

EPIDEMIOLOGY AND PATHOGENESIS

H. pylori is one of the most prevalent infections worldwide. In developed countries infection rates rise from

Notes

less than 10% in the first decade of life to about 50% in the fourth decade. It is believed that the infection is transmitted by the oral–oral or faecal–oral route and hence is most common in circumstances of overcrowding in the family home. In the underdeveloped world infection rates generally exceed 70% by the second decade. Because transmission of diseases by these routes are features of youth, it is believed that infection with *H. pylori* demonstrates a cohort phenomenon with infection being contracted early in life and then persisting. In the developed world it is apparent that it is unusual to contract infection as an adult. Thus infection rates may drop naturally as the members of the high-prevalence age groups die.

The organism survives in a particular environment which protects it from destruction. It lives below the mucus layer but on the surface of gastric mucosal cells. Here it provokes an inflammatory and immune response which, unaided, seems incapable of clearing the organism. It does not seem to survive on other types of mucosa and hence is found in sites other than the stomach only when ectopic gastric mucosa is present. Gastric metaplasia is common in the duodenum and possibly reflects genetic, environmental, and physiologic factors which may vary from one individual to another; increased acid secretion, long known to be associated with duodenal ulcer, promotes gastric metaplastic change in the duodenum. Thus the hypothesis has developed that in certain individuals gastric metaplasia in the duodenum allows colonization with *H. pylori* (spread from its usual home of gastric antrum) with subsequent ulceration. In addition there is evidence that in such people the gastric response

Notes

to food is to produce higher than normal levels of acid secretion. Thus *H. pylori* may promote the gastric metaplasia through gastric hypersecretion in some. However, in others gastric ulcer develops and acid secretion in such people is normal to low. The mechanism of ulceration here is more difficult to explain.

PRESENTATION

In general *H. pylori* infection goes unnoticed until some other pathology develops which produces symptoms. There is no doubt that in dyspepsia *Helicobacter* infection is found more commonly than in people without symptoms. While this demonstrates its involvement in producing symptoms or symptomatic disease, it is clear that it does not produce symptoms in a large proportion of infected patients and it is unclear whether *H. pylori* is the cause of symptoms in the remainder. It has been reported that acute infection in adults produces a short illness of abdominal discomfort, malaise, and nausea which may be associated with hypochlorhydria. However, acute infection in adults is thought to be rare and there is presently no means of identifying acute infection in children. Thus *H. pylori* is usually diagnosed when patients present with dyspepsia or during endoscopy.

MANAGEMENT

We advise treatment to eliminate *H. pylori* in all patients with duodenal and gastric ulcer where the organism is present. This advice is based on evidence of benefit in that ulcer recurrence is extremely unusual following

Notes

successful eradication. There is considerable interest in attempting to eliminate the infection in dyspeptics before investigation, or in ulcer-negative dyspepsia, but at present there are few data to suggest that benefit ensues. Present treatment regimens are complex and have significant side-effects (see *2.1.8 Anti-*Helicobacter pylori *Treatment*) and we would not change our advice until it becomes clear that either treatment is completely safe, cheap, and simple or that it provides a substantial benefit to patients and health services. We believe that *H. pylori* should be shown to be present before treatment, either by serologic testing in untreated patients and by endoscopic methods or urea breath-testing in others. This area of therapy is likely to change substantially in the next decade and up-to-date reviews are recommended.

The most successful therapeutic regimens involve three drugs. One contains either bismuth or an anti-secretory agent, and the other two are standard antibiotics. Modern treatment schedules are simpler but all involve a major effort on behalf of the patient. Compliance has been shown to be the most important determinant of successful treatment. In clinical trials eradication rates of 90% and above should be expected, although in practice treatment results are likely to be less successful as compliance drops off. Treatment durations of 1 week seem adequate with the present best regimens. Treatment regimens containing metronidazole (or tinidazole) and clarithromycin depend to a limited extent on the prevalence of bacterial resistance to these antibiotics. As adult to adult spread of the organism is rare it is unlikely that more resistance will develop in the population through use of these antibiotics for

Notes

Helicobacter eradication. However, use of these agents singly for other conditions may be associated with increased resistance rates and therefore the treatment regimens suggested in 1997 may not be appropriate for 2000.

1.2.7

Stress Ulceration

Stress ulcers are acute superficial ulcers that occur predominantly in the stomach and are a recognized feature of severe physical stress, burns, and trauma.

EPIDEMIOLOGY AND PATHOLOGY

The pathophysiology is poorly understood but may be related to mucosal hypoxia or poor perfusion. There is no evidence that excessive acid secretion is a provocation and, when measured, gastric pH may be higher than normal in such patients. Modern intensive care seems to have reduced the frequency of problems from stress ulceration and it is not clear whether prophylactic therapy has played a part in this. Devastating gastric bleeding, sometimes requiring total gastrectomy, was a well recognized occurrence due to stress ulcers.

PRESENTATION

Gastric bleeding on an intensive care unit in a patient with severe burns or head trauma is likely to be due to stress ulceration.

Notes

INVESTIGATION

The diagnosis is dependent on endoscopy, although the emphasis is on prevention.

MANAGEMENT

Prophylaxis is believed to be important although convincing evidence is generally lacking. Three forms of treatment have been applied: *regular antacid, H_2-receptor antagonists* and *sucralphate*. The clinical doses are as for treatment of peptic ulcer (see *1.2.4 Gastric Ulcer*) except that sucralphate should be given as the suspension, 1 g every 4 hours to a maximum of 8 g daily, and the H_2-receptor antagonists can be given by intravenous bolus or by continuous infusion. These latter drugs have been blamed for causing hospital-acquired infection of the lungs through reducing the natural gastric bactericidal activity due to acid. Sucralphate is not believed to be associated with such nosocomial pneumonia, although evidence is sparse in either case.

1.2.8

Duodenitis

DEFINITION

Duodenitis is a histologic diagnosis akin to gastritis (see *1.2.3*). Many endoscopists also report a macroscopic abnormality of reddening with or without tiny ulcers or erosions as duodenitis. The correlation between such reports and histologic findings is poor.

Notes

EPIDEMIOLOGY AND PATHOLOGY

Duodenitis is a relatively common finding during the investigation of dyspepsia, although it may not be the cause of the symptoms. The etiology of the inflammation is generally unknown (nonspecific duodenitis), although there is an association with gastric metaplasia and *H. pylori*. It is possibly also produced by other infections like Giardia, tuberculosis, cryptosporidia and Strongyloides, but in the West these problems are rare.

PRESENTATION

Duodenitis is discovered during endoscopy, usually for dyspepsia. It may not be the cause of the patient's symptoms.

MANAGEMENT

Treatment is difficult and few clinical trials of drugs for duodenitis have been published. Many treat the condition as if for duodenal ulcer (see *1.2.5*) but it possibly behaves differently. Symptomatic treatment with *antacids* and *H_2-receptor antagonists* may be worth trying. Repeat endoscopy is not required.

1.2.9

Gastric Cancer

Stomach cancer presents late and is commonly incurable.

Notes

EPIDEMIOLOGY AND PATHOLOGY

Cure is so rare in most countries that gastric cancer death is an accepted measure of incidence. The disease frequency varies between countries: Japan has an annual mortality rate six times that in the United States. Incidence varies substantially even within a country. The disease is more common in men, and affects old people most. The frequency of gastric cancer is decreasing throughout the world, although increasing numbers of old people make this difficult to believe at times. It is probable that proximal gastric cancer affecting the upper part of the stomach is decreasing less than antral cancer, and it may even be increasing like oesophageal adenocarcinoma. Blood group A seems protective but the disease is more frequently found in first-degree relatives. It is postulated that gastric cancer progresses from gastritis with or without intestinal metaplasia and atrophy to dysplasia. *H. pylori* is the commonest international cause of gastritis and has been shown in epidemiologic surveys to be associated with development of gastric cancer. Other etiological postulates include diets deficient in fresh vegetables and vitamin C, and those replete with salt and *N*-nitrosamines. The cancers are predominantly adenocarcinoma and may be reported as intestinal or diffuse, expanding or infiltrative, as papillary, mucinous, signet ring, or tubular, among many different classifications.

PRESENTATION

Dyspepsia is a feature, at some stage, of most cases. There is nothing specific about the indigestion of gastric

Notes

cancer. Gastric ulcer can be coincident and, when malignant, may be indistinguishable macroscopically from a benign ulcer. Thus all ulcers seen endoscopically should be biopsied and samples for cytology taken. An epigastric mass and severe weight loss are suggestive of more advanced, and usually incurable, disease. Very advanced disease may present with massive hepatomegaly and even ascites.

INVESTIGATIONS

Upper gastrointestinal endoscopy is the single most important investigation. It offers the opportunity to assess intragastric site and size, and to obtain a histological diagnosis. Barium meal radiography also demonstrates most cancers but can not always distinguish between benign and malignant mucosal disease. Diagnosis should not be delayed when gastric cancer is suspected because only lesions that are small and relatively noninvasive are curable.

MANAGEMENT

The only treatment that could potentially cure the disease is surgical removal. One trial has suggested that long-term *cimetidine* can prolong survival in patients with extensive disease and other antisecretory agents may usefully control symptoms.

Notes

1.2.10

Gastric Lymphoma

EPIDEMIOLOGY AND PATHOLOGY

Primary gastric nonHodgkin's lymphoma is rare at about 1–3% of all gastric malignancy. It is more common in men and presents in the late 50s and 60s. It can be found as a large mass, as a well circumscribed ulcer, and as diffuse ulceration. When the cells are similar in appearance to Peyer's patches, it is usually a low-grade B-cell tumour and has been termed MALT lymphoma (mucosa-associated lymphoid tissue). In such cases the B cells all derive from the same clone and thus it can be distinguished from lymphoid infiltration seen with gastritis. These cases are frequently associated with *H. pylori* infection (see *1.2.6*) and carry a relatively good prognosis. High-grade MALT lymphoma is less responsive. It is not clear whether these malignancies are similar to nodal nonHodgkin's lymphoma. Gastric lymphoma is associated with immunodeficiency syndromes.

PRESENTATION

Epigastric pain is the prominent symptom but may be indistinguishable from symptoms of other causes of dyspepsia. Weight loss and vomiting ensue as the tumour advances.

INVESTIGATION

Upper gastrointestinal endoscopy will usually make the diagnosis but sometimes biopsies are inconclusive if the

Notes

disease is deep to the mucosa. A biopsy urease test for *H. pylori* should be taken from a macroscopically normal-looking area in the antrum if possible, and an attempt should also be made to identify the organisms microscopically.

MANAGEMENT

Surgery is the main mode of treatment for localized disease but may be less appropriate for high-grade tumours with spread. In such cases oncologic support with chemotherapy should be sought. When *H. pylori* is identified, eradication (see *2.1.8 Anti-*Helicobacter pylori *Treatment*) should be attempted as early studies show complete tumour regression in some cases of low-grade MALT lymphoma. It is too soon to know which patients may respond and whether that response is long lasting, but little harm can come from attempting to treat the organism. In diffuse cases of MALT lymphoma, *H. pylori* eradication and endoscopic surveillance is probably first-line therapy.

1.2.11

Gastric Polyps and Benign Tumours

EPIDEMIOLOGY AND PATHOLOGY

Gastric polyps are found in 1–3% of routine gastroscopies. They are most commonly hyperplastic and of little consequence. Adenomatous polyps may have some malignant potential, but it is not agreed how likely

Notes

malignant change is. Leiomyoma is also a relatively common finding and can ulcerate on the surface giving characteristic radiologic and endoscopic features. Multiple gastric polyps (with definite malignant potential) occur in familial polyposis, and hamartomas may be found in Peutz–Jeghers syndrome and in neurofibromatosis. Rarely, polypoid lesions arise from heterotopic pancreatic tissue or ectopic Brunner's glands. Multiple polyps are occasionally seen in pernicious anaemia or atrophic gastritis due to enterochromaffin-like carcinoids.

PRESENTATION

It is likely that most gastric polyps are incidental findings, although most patients are under investigation for dyspepsia so it is possible that the polyps are symptomatic. They can bleed, presenting acutely (particularly leiomyomata) or with iron deficiency anaemia.

MANAGEMENT

It is unusual to have to resort to surgical removal except for large lesions associated with bleeding. Pedunculated lesions can safely be removed endoscopically allowing full histologic analysis and this is advisable whenever feasible. Tiny lesions should be biopsied to exclude early gastric malignancy. No particular drug therapy is required.

General Gastrointestinal Conditions and Issues

1.3.1

Vomiting

Vomiting is a symptom associated with a multitude of other conditions including gastrointestinal, metabolic, central nervous, and psychologic disorders. It is commonly provoked by cytotoxic drug therapies and other therapeutic agents and may be secondary to severe pain of any cause. Thus management depends importantly on identification of an underlying cause, treatment of which may make antiemetic therapy unnecessary.

PATHOGENESIS

Elucidation of the cause is the single most useful "therapy" in the assessment of vomiting. Vomiting may be a symptom of gastrointestinal disease: ulcers, esophagitis, gastritis and duodenitis, hiatus hernia, gallstones, pancreatitis, hepatitis, intestinal obstruction, gastric cancer, and gastroenteritis. Most of these conditions require specific treatment. It should be remembered, however, that vomiting can be the presenting feature of pregnancy, vestibular problems, and raised intracranial pressure, and is frequently associated with intracranial haemorrhage, migraine, and febrile illnesses in children. Pain itself can provoke vomiting irrespective of the cause; thus vomiting with renal colic or myocardial infarction is well recognized. Medication is another prominent cause of nausea and vomiting, notably digoxin, opiates, erythromycin, and anaesthetic agents, amongst many. Metabolic disturbance, particularly hypercalcemia, is often associated with vomiting.

Notes

As vomiting can be produced by so many different mechanisms its understanding is limited. Therapeutic intervention is aimed at raising the central nervous vomiting threshold at the chemoreceptor trigger-zone, increasing and decreasing intestinal and gastric motility, and inhibiting peripheral serotonin activity.

INVESTIGATIONS

These depend on clinical circumstances and will frequently include a biochemical assessment, endoscopy, ultrasonography of the gallbladder, and more specific radiology of the abdomen and head when clinically appropriate.

MANAGEMENT

The underlying cause should be sought and treated. Where symptomatic therapy is still required the agents discussed below can be considered. Details of these drugs are not given in *Section B*.

Selective 5-hydroxytryptamine antagonists

The selective 5-hydroxytryptamine ($5\text{-}HT_3$ serotonin) antagonists (ondansetron, granisetron, and tropisetron) are the most effective and most expensive agents. They act on acetylcholine release in the gastrointestinal tract. They are particularly useful in patients with such severe vomiting that oral agents are unreasonable or where cheaper oral agents are ineffective. The main role for these agents is in treating the unwanted effects of

Notes

chemotherapy and radiotherapy. Oncologic advice should be taken if these agents are being considered. They can be given by the enteral or parenteral route.

Anticholinergics

Hyoscine (scopolamine) is effective if vomiting is not too severe. Anticholinergic side-effects and drowsiness limit its usefulness. A transcutaneous osmotic pump delivering consistent low-dose scopolamine is available for long-duration effect.

Histamine H_1-receptor antagonists

Cyclizine is one of many used with some effect in motion sickness and labyrinthine disorders, and to deal with the unwanted nausea associated with opiates. Drowsiness and mild anticholinergic effects are not uncommon. Excitation can occur in children.

Phenothiazines

Prochlorperazine is one of many. It is effective in the same indications as the antihistamines and may share some of the unwanted effects, as phenothiazines often have some antihistamine and anticholinergic activity. Extrapyramidal reactions are well recognized.

Metoclopramide

A dopamine antagonist, like the phenothiazines, it is thought to inhibit the chemoreceptor trigger zone. It also has a peripheral effect stimulating gastric emptying. It is effective only in standard doses (10 mg) in mild nausea

Notes

and vomiting but has been used in high dose for chemotherapy-induced vomiting. Extrapyramidal effects including tardive dyskinesia are well recognized.

Domperidone

Domperidone is similar to metoclopramide without any central effects, so tardive dyskinesia is less likely. Oral preparations only are used for mild nausea.

1.3.2

Gastrointestinal Bleeding

This section covers a condition that results from many different causes. It should be used in conjunction with sections covering the specific disease wherever mentioned.

Gastrointestinal blood loss may be acute and obvious leading to hypovolemia, or it may be occult leading to anaemia. It is useful to define bleeding by broad site (upper and lower intestine) as it is usually simple to distinguish the two clinically.

1.3.2.1

UPPER GASTROINTESTINAL BLEEDING

EPIDEMIOLOGY AND PATHOLOGY

Patients with haematemesis and/or melena are bleeding from one of the conditions shown in *Table 1*. Peptic ulcer bleeding accounts for approximately half the cases and

Notes

Table 1 Causes of upper and lower gastrointestinal bleeding

Cause	Percentage
Upper	
Duodenal ulcer	22–30
Gastric ulcer	14–25
Mallory–Weiss tear	4–23
Oesophagitis	<12
Acute gastric erosions	<7
Oesophageal varices	3–20
Gastric cancer	1–3
Other diagnosis	<30
No clear diagnosis	3–27
Lower	
Angiodysplasia	10
Diverticular disease	80
Haemorrhoids Ulcerative or Crohn's colitis Polyps Cancer Ischaemic colitis Meckel's diverticulum Colonic varices	20

an association with nonsteroidal anti-inflammatory drugs (NSAIDs) is found in 40–60% of these. It is not known what other host factors provoke bleeding, although the site of the ulcer in relation to vessels is clearly important. There are 100 admissions per 100 000 population annually for gastrointestinal bleeding, and although data collection has been hampered by changes in methods of recording and classification it is clear that admissions are decreasing in the UK and other European

Notes

countries. This overall reduction is associated with an increase in admissions for peptic ulcer amongst the elderly, particularly women, some of which can be explained by NSAID use. All NSAIDs are implicated, although some (piroxicam and indomethacin) appear more likely to be associated with bleeding than others (ibuprofen), and the risk associated with low-dose aspirin used for cardiovascular protection is measurable but low. All other causes of upper gastrointestinal bleeding are relatively rare in comparison, Mallory–Weiss tears being more common in young men following alcoholic binges. Oesophagitis (see *1.1.1 Oesophageal Reflux Disease*) leading to overt bleeding is a feature of the elderly. Oesophageal varices are an important if infrequent cause of gastrointestinal bleeding (see *1.5.1 Variceal Bleeding*). It is important to realize also that in a proportion of cases no clear diagnosis is made despite rapid investigation.

PRESENTATION

Patients present with either haematemesis or melena, or a combination of the two. There is some evidence to suggest that the chances of rebleeding are greatest in those presenting with haematemesis. A typical history of retching followed by bright red haematemesis is a useful indicant of Mallory–Weiss tears. Recent use of NSAIDs, a past history of peptic ulcer, and typical indigestion may also help in diagnosis. Alcohol abuse may also raise the suspicion of oesophageal varices. The volume of vomit described by the patient is, in our opinion, useless in assessment of severity. Much better is a sense of dizziness

Notes

or actual collapse. The colour of the vomit may be helpful in that "coffee grounds" rarely represent severe acute bleeding and may suggest small amounts of mucosal oozing while clots of dark red blood suggest substantial bleeding. Bleeding from the upper gastrointestinal tract associated with bright red rectal bleeding is always associated with hypotension and it is a safe assumption that patients presenting with bright red rectal bleeding who have no evidence of hypovolemia are bleeding from the lower gastrointestinal tract.

INVESTIGATIONS

Clinical measurements come first. Is there evidence of hypovolemia from tachycardia or postural drop in blood pressure? Can you confirm evidence of bleeding by inspecting stool or vomit and, if not, does a rectal examination demonstrate melena? The baseline haemoglobin level is useful but is not a measure of severity of bleeding as it can take 12–24 hours to drop after haemodilution despite substantial haemorrhage. The blood urea is commonly raised after substantial upper gastrointestinal bleeding which provides a large protein load to the gut. The serum creatinine level should be normal unless there is underlying coincidental renal disease.

Endoscopy is the most useful diagnostic investigation, but should be performed by the most experienced endoscopist available. Apart from probably identifying the source of blood loss, endoscopists can apply therapy, injecting ulcers with visible vessels and varices with sclerosant, adrenaline, or alcohol. Barium meal examinations are a poor substitute because blood clot may

Notes

obscure adequate interpretation and therapy can not be applied.

MANAGEMENT

The management of oesophageal varices is dealt with separately. The management of gastrointestinal bleeding is aided by the use of guidelines, which should be available to all doctors. Those provided by the Royal College of Physicians of London are helpful. The mortality rate associated with gastrointestinal bleeding varies from hospital to hospital within the same groups of patients, and guidelines should be able to standardize management and hence outcome. Maintenance of a normal haemodynamic state is the aim of therapy. If bleeding does not stop spontaneously, it should be clear clinically and measures taken to stem the bleeding should be taken, whether endoscopic or surgical. Thus the decision about when to intervene physically must be taken rationally. Patients may die from surgical intervention but by the same token they are at significant risk if surgical intervention is delayed too long. Older patients bleeding from peptic ulcer do worst if surgery is delayed too long. *Patients aged over 60 years should be submitted for surgery if they have one clinical rebleed from peptic ulceration in hospital or require more than 4 units of blood in 24 hours to maintain haemodynamic stability or more than 8 units overall. Patients with peptic ulcer aged under 60 years are submitted for surgery with two episodes of rebleeding, or the requirement for 8 units of blood over 24 hours to maintain blood pressure. All patients with spurting vessels at endoscopy despite endoscopic therapy are referred for urgent*

Notes

surgery. This protocol has been associated with low mortality rates of 2–8% depending on age, and limits unnecessary surgery.

Pharmacologic intervention

There are a number of small trials which suggest that antisecretory agents are beneficial, but the two largest studies were unable to show that either intravenous *omeprazole* or *famotidine* reduced rebleeding, surgery, or mortality. Antisecretory therapy is therefore not recommended. The use of the antifibrinolytic agent tranexamic acid has been associated with improved outcome. It can be given orally or intravenously starting from the time of admission. *Somatostatin* or an analogue has been shown to help in bleeding from oesophageal varices but data demonstrating benefit in other circumstances are less convincing.

Endoscopic intervention

Injection of sclerosant substances, alcohol, adrenaline, and even water around the base of a visible vessel or around oozing has been shown to stop bleeding. The application of heat by electrodes or laser beam also stops bleeding and all means are associated with reduced rebleeding. One controlled study has clearly demonstrated that endoscopic therapy can be beneficial. It should be applied whenever bleeding or nonbleeding vessels are seen during endoscopy for acute haemorrhage. However, the guidelines regarding surgery should be adhered to if endoscopic therapy is unsuccessful.

Notes

Subsequent treatment

Where ulcers have been found treatment should follow usual recommendations with eradication of *Helicobacter pylori* whenever present (see *2.1.8 Anti-*Helicobacter pylori *Treatment*). In patients who present with bleeding when taking NSAIDs, long-term therapy should be considered if the NSAID has to be continued. There is evidence that *misoprostol* can prevent recurrent peptic ulcer complications from NSAIDs. *Omeprazole* has also been demonstrated to be better than ranitidine in preventing recurrent gastric or duodenal ulcer related to continued NSAIDs. Iron supplementation to replace stores is sensible for all patients but they should be warned that stool colour will change to dark greeny black.

1.3.2.2

LOWER GASTROINTESTINAL BLEEDING

PATHOLOGY

The causes of acute lower gastrointestinal bleeding are shown in *Table 1*.

PRESENTATION

Bleeding from the lower gastrointestinal tract is rarely as profuse as upper gastrointestinal bleeding. The stool contains red or plum-coloured blood which distresses the patient but does not commonly produce haemodynamic

Notes

instability. Occasionally bleeding from the caecum can present with melena and may be difficult to distinguish from upper gastrointestinal blood loss.

INVESTIGATIONS

Sigmoidoscopy and proctoscopy are the most important investigations. These simple tests will immediately diagnose colitis, haemorrhoids, rectal and sigmoid polyps, and cancer. Angiodysplasia requires a well prepared bowel and colonoscopy, but can be shown in many cases by angiography of excellent quality. Diverticular disease and often the source of bleeding may be identified by colonoscopy, which is therefore the investigation of choice. It can be performed as an emergency following limited preparation when continued bleeding compromises the clinical state. Technetium pertechnetate scans, barium enema, and angiography have to be considered in difficult cases with continuing bleeding.

MANAGEMENT

Individual conditions are all dealt with elsewhere. Pharmacologic intervention is not routine.

1.3.3

Nutritional Support

The optimal management of many disease states depends on appropriate nutritional support. Over recent

Notes

decades, this has evolved from "hyperalimentation" to more precise patient-specific feeding based on an understanding of the physiology and metabolism of different disease states. The aim is to correct malnutrition or prevent nutritional depletion in order to optimize patient recovery.

A complete coverage of enteral and parenteral nutrition is beyond the scope of this book. Thus this section will primarily cover issues related to nutritional assessment, nutritional requirements, and the method of nutritional support.

INDICATIONS

The indications for nutritional support are:

1 Severe malnutrition
2 An adequate oral intake not expected for 3–5 days in significantly malnourished patients, 5–8 days in previously well nourished patients, or 2–3 days in patients in intensive care.

ASSESSMENT OF NUTRITIONAL STATUS

A wide variety of methods is used to assess nutritional status. The most suitable combine clinical assessment with objective measures. Clinically important aspects to consider are outlined in *Table 2*.

Blood parameters that may indicate malnutrition include anaemia (due to iron or folate or both), lymphocytopenia, hypoalbuminemia, low serum transferrin and prealbumin levels, and vitamin deficiency (particularly white cell vitamin C and red cell B_2) (*Table 3*).

Notes

Table 2 Clinical indicators of risk of malnutrition

Indicator	Finding
Weight loss	Loss in preceding 6 months (5–10% "potentially significant", >10% "definitely significant") and the change in the preceding 2 weeks (increased, no change, decreased)
Dietary intake	Duration and degree of reduced dietary intake
Gastrointestinal symptoms	Anorexia, nausea, vomiting, diarrhoea for >2 weeks
Functional capacity	Duration and degree of reduced functional capacity (bedridden > ambulatory > working suboptimally)
Physical signs	Loss of subcutaneous fat, muscle wasting, peripheral oedema, ascites
Disease	Metabolic demand of the disease state

From Detsky AS, McLaughlin JR, Baker JP, et al. *Journal of Parenteral and Enteral Nutrition* 1985; **11**: 8–13.

1.3

Table 3 Assessment of blood parameters

Assessment	Degree of malnutrition		
	Normal	Moderate	Severe
Serum albumin ($g\ l^{-1}$)	35–50	21–30	<21
Serum transferrin ($g\ l^{-1}$)	200–400	100–150	<100
Serum prealbumin ($mg\ l^{-1}$)	>170	110–150	<110
Total lymphocyte count ($10^6\ l^{-1}$)	1.8–3.0	0.8–1.2	<0.8

Notes

Serum prealbumin may be one of the most practical of these measures of malnutrition because it is a protein with an easily measured rapid turnover (half-life < 2 days) that is prognostically valuable in assessing and monitoring patients (*Table* 4.). An increase in prealbumin concentration of 10 $mg\,l^{-1}\,day^{-1}$ is said to reflect anabolism and an improvement of less than 40 $mg\,l^{-1}$ per week is a poor response.

Most clinicians use a combination of the above subjective and objective measures to grade their patients as being well nourished, moderately (or suspected of being) malnourished, or severely malnourished. This gives a reliable indication of the need for nutritional support. In addition, the likelihood of support being needed increases with age (especially in patients aged over 40 years) and if malignant disease (especially gastrointestinal) is present.

NUTRITIONAL SUPPORT

Enteral nutritional support is preferred to parenteral support because it is more physiologic, less invasive, safer, and much less expensive. The main absolute

Table 4 Risk assessment using prealbumin

Prealbumin level ($mg\,l^{-1}$)*	**Risk level**
< 50	Poor prognosis
50–109	Significant risk, aggressive nutritional support indicated
110–150	Increased risk, monitor status carefully

**Normal range 170–420 mg* l^{-1}.

(Bernstein L, et al. Nutrition 1995; **11**: 169–171)

Notes

contraindication to enteral feeding is mechanical obstruction. Other indications for parenteral support are outlined in *Table 5*. Severe diarrhoea, gastric stasis, enteric fistulae, and intestinal dysmotility may provide special challenges to enteral feeding, but are not necessarily contraindications. Occasionally enteral feeds may need to be supplemented with parenteral nutrition.

MANAGEMENT

The types of enteral formula and their administration are discussed under *Enteral Nutritional Solutions* (see 2.2.7). Further consideration of parenteral nutrition is not appropriate for this text.

Table 5 Indications for parenteral nutritional support

Main indications	Possible indications (if enteral feeding too difficult or inadequate)
Mechanical gastrointestinal tract obstruction	Prolonged gut dysmotility (ileus, gastroparesis)
Massive bowel resection	Enteric fistulae (especially proximal fistulae)
Severe pancreatitis	Severe diarrhoea
Pancreatitis with complications	Moderate pancreatitis
Postpancreatic surgery	Severe trauma, burns
Failed enteral feeding	Adjunct to chemotherapy Acute renal failure, hepatic failure Other catabolic states

Notes

The choice of an enteral formula is dependent on an individual's requirements. This needs primarily to take into account daily calorie, protein, and fluid requirements. Additional consideration should be given to the composition of nonprotein calories and replacement of excess loss or deficiencies of electrolytes, vitamins, and trace elements.

Calorie requirements

General calorie requirements can be estimated using the values in *Table 6*.

A more precise way of determining the resting energy expenditure is indirect calorimetry. This, however, is often not available. Alternatively energy requirement (ER) can be estimated from the resting energy expenditure (REE), based on the Harris–Benedict equation, with adjustment for activity and stress.

$$\text{REE (males) (kcal day}^{-1}) = 66.5 + [13.8 \times \text{wt (kg)}] + [5 \times \text{ht (cm)}] - [6.8 \times \text{age (yrs)}]$$

$$\text{REE (females) (kcal day}^{-1}) = 65.5 + [9.6 \times \text{wt (kg)}] + [1.8 \times \text{ht (cm)}] - [4.7 \times \text{age (yrs)}]$$

$$\text{ER} = \text{REE} \times \text{activity factor} \times \text{stress factor}$$

Table 6 General calorie requirements

Condition	Requirement (kcal kg^{-1} day^{-1})
Normal maintenance or elective surgery	25
Trauma, acute pancreatitis, inflammatory bowel disease	30
Sepsis, minor burns	35
Major burns, severe trauma	40

Notes

Activity factor: 1.25 (ambulatory)
Stress factor: 1.2 (minor operation), 1.35 (trauma), 1.6 (sepsis), 2.1 (burns)

In most circumstances the ER overestimates actual needs. Excessive caloric replacement may actually be harmful with an increased risk of nosocomial infection. Thus caloric replacement approximating the result of the Harris–Benedict equation without adjustments is usually sufficient.

Protein requirements

The daily protein requirement for a healthy adult is 0.8–1.0 g per kg body weight. In hypermetabolic states, as in sepsis or cancer, the daily protein requirement increases (*Table 7*).

Table 7 Protein requirements

Status	**Estimated requirement (g kg^{-1})**
Normal (adult)	0.8–1.0
Noncatabolic malnourished	1.2–1.5
Moderate stress (infection, fracture, surgery)	1.0–2.0
Severe stress (burns, multiple fracture)	2.0–2.5
Renal disease	
Uremic no dialysis	0.6
Haemodialysis	1.0–1.2
Chronic ambulatory peritoneal dialysis	1.2–1.5
Liver disease with encephalopathy	0.6

Notes

Fluid requirements

Most adults drink about 1000–1500 ml of liquids per day. About 1000 ml per day also comes from the ingestion of solid food. Additional fluids may be required to replace abnormal losses associated with fever, excessive perspiration, fistula and wound drainage, vomiting, and diarrhoea (*Table 8*). *Table 9* shows the fluid requirements of adult and pediatric patients.

Nonprotein caloric requirements

There is uncertainty regarding the optimal proportion of calories provided by carbohydrate or fat in the diet. Generally at least 30–40% should be provided by fat. The diet should also include adequate amounts of vitamins, minerals, and electrolytes to meet the Recommended Dietary Allowances. Excess electrolyte losses also need replacement.

Table 8 Enteric fluid volumes and electrolytes

Enteric secretion	Volume ($l\,day^{-1}$)	Electrolytes ($mmol\,l^{-1}$)			
		Na	K	Cl	HCO_3
Saliva	1–2	10	30	10	30
Gastric juice	2	60	9	90	0
Pancreatic fluid	?	130	5	75	90
Bile	2–3	150	10	90	70
Small bowel	1	100	5	100	20
Colon	Variable	40	100	15	60

Notes

Table 9 Baseline daily fluid requirements of adult and pediatric patients

Patient group	Fluid requirement
Children (< 16 years)	
0.5–3 kg	120 ml kg^{-1}
3–10 kg	100 ml kg^{-1}
10–20 kg	1000 ml + 50 ml kg^{-1} for each kg over 10 kg
> 20 kg	1500 ml + 20 ml kg^{-1} for each kg over 20 kg
Adults	
Young active (16–30 years)	40 ml kg^{-1}
Average adult (25–55 years)	35 ml kg^{-1}
Older patients (56–65 years)	30 ml kg^{-1}
Elderly (> 65 years)	25 ml kg^{-1}

1.3.4

Endoscopy – Antibiotic Prophylaxis

Whether or not antibiotic prophylaxis of serious infection, such as infective endocarditis, is appropriate will depend both on a patient's individual risk and on the risk of the endoscopic procedure. *Table 10* outlines when antibiotic prophylaxis is recommended.

There are many similar effective prophylactic regimens. *Table 11* shows one that is suitable for most patients. Exceptions may include those with renal impairment or clinical infection. If there is doubt about the appropriateness of the regimen then an infectious diseases physician should be consulted.

Notes

1.3

Table 10 Need for antibiotic prophylaxis

Increased patient risk	Increased procedural risk
Previous endocarditis	All endoscopic procedures
Prosthetic heart valve arteriovenous shunt, indwelling vascular device	All endoscopic procedures with the exception of simple diagnostic EGD
Seriously impaired immune function	Colonoscopy or any other procedure with tissue disruption, including simple EGD if severe mucositis
Bile duct obstruction	ERCP
Intrinsic infective foci	Procedure, irrespective of type, adjacent to infective foci Percutaneous endoscopic gastrostomy (PEG) or jejunostomy (PEJ)

EGD, oesophagogastroduodenoscopy; ERCP, – endoscopic retrograde cholangiopancreatography.

Table 11 Antibiotic regimens for patients having endoscopy

	Antiobiotic	Route of administration
Standard		
Before procedure	Ampicillin 1 g (50 mg kg^{-1} up to adult dose) and gentamicin 1.5 mg kg^{-1} (2.5 mg kg^{-1}, maximum dose 80 mg)	Intravenously just before procedure or intramuscularly 30 min beforehand
After procedure	Ampicillin or amoxycillin 500 mg (25 mg kg^{-1} up to adult dose)	Intravenously or orally 6 hours after procedure
Penicillin allergy	Vancomycin 1 g (20 mg kg^{-1} up to adult dose) and gentamicin (as above)	Intravenously, slowly, just before procedure

Small and Large Intestine

1.4.1

Overview of Infectious Diarrhoea

Infections (especially viral and bacterial) are the most common cause of acute diarrhoea, and may cause chronic diarrhoea (*Table 12*).

PRESENTATION

1.4

The area of bowel affected may be suggested by the character of the stool and by the features of accompanying pain. Small bowel diarrhoea is likely to be large in volume, watery, offensive, light in colour, free of blood, and contain undigested food particles. Accompanying pain is often colicky and localized to the periumbilical region or right iliac fossa. Large bowel diarrhoea may be small in volume. The faeces are usually soft and dark in colour, and may contain mucus and blood (dysentery). Pain may be suprapubic and is usually relieved by defecation. There is considerable overlap.

INVESTIGATIONS

In most instances the specific diagnosis of a gastrointestinal infection depends on finding the causative agent in a faecal specimen. Faecal specimens should be obtained as early as possible especially before any antimicrobial treatment has commenced.

A mild, self-limited course is usual and neither a specific diagnosis nor treatment is required in most instances. Patients who benefit from further investigation have either a severe or dysenteric illness, or a prolonged

Notes

Table 12 Classification of the causes of diarrhoea

Acute diarrhoea (<3 weeks' duration)
Infective
Food poisoning
Drugs, including antibiotics and food additives
Faecal impaction
Pelvic inflammation
Heavy metal poisoning (tin, zinc, copper, cadmium)
Traveller's diarrhoea
Diarrhoea in a homosexual without HIV infection
Diarrhoea with HIV infection
Chronic recurrent diarrhoea
Irritable bowel syndrome
Drugs, including antibiotics and food additives
Inflammatory bowel disease
Parasitic and fungal infections
Colonic cancer
Diverticulitis
Watery diarrhoea–colitis syndrome
Malabsorption or maldigestion
Secretory diarrhoea
Laxative abuse
Faecal impaction
Heavy metal poisoning
Incontinence
Sphincter dysfunction
Causes of chronic diarrhoea as above

Italics indicate topics discussed in Section 1.4. HIV, human immunodeficiency virus.

course. A high concentration of faecal leucocytes on a smear suggests an invasive pathogen, or inflammatory bowel disease (*Table 13*). Severe dysentery may be difficult to distinguish from acute ulcerative colitis and

Notes

Table 13 Infectious diarrhoea and faecal leucocytes

Faecal leucocytes	No faecal leucocytes
Campylobacter	Viral
Shigella	*Salmonella*
Enteroinvasive *Escherichia coli*	*C. difficile*
Enterohemorrhagic *E. coli*	Food poisoning
	Yersinia
Viral (uncommon)	*Aeromonas*
Yersinia (rare)	*Giardia lamblia*
Salmonella (rare)	*E. histolytica*
Clostridium difficile (rare)	Enterotoxigenic *E. coli*
Entamoeba histolytica (rare)	Enteropathogenic *E. coli*
Aeromonas (rare)	*V. parahemolyticus*
Vibrio parahemolyticus (rare)	*Vibrio cholerae**

* *Geographically limited.*

1.4

faecal cultures demonstrate a cause in only 50%. Early endoscopic biopsies may help to distinguish between infective colitis and ulcerative colitis.

MANAGEMENT

Adequate rehydration and continued hydration is the mainstay of treatment. Oral rehydration is appropriate if the degree of dehydration is less than 10% (see 2.2.2 *Oral Rehydration Solutions*). If there is severe dehydration then replacement should primarily be with intravenous fluids. The state of hydration should be reassessed after 4–6 hours and, if the patient is rehydrated, ongoing fluid replacement should be sufficient to replace ongoing losses (diarrhoea, vomiting, urinary and insensible losses).

Notes

After adequate rehydration, the patient should be allowed to eat. Nutrition at an early stage is important for calorie intake and improves outcome. In infants, a full-strength, lactose-free formula given immediately after rehydration reduces stool volume and the duration of diarrhoea more than delaying feeding. Lactose malabsorption is a common sequel, especially after viral diarrhoea, but nevertheless most infants tolerate breast-feeding together with oral rehydration solutions. Breast-feeding is associated with a better outcome than other means of nutritional support.

The food intake in older children and adults should be low in simple sugars (except glucose) and fat, and free from caffeine or methylxanthine. Aerated soft drinks, fruit juices, coffee, cocoa, strong tea, and fried foods should be avoided.

Antidiarrhoeals (see *2.2.1*) may relieve acute diarrhoea of varying causes. A major use is in "traveller's diarrhoea" (see *1.4.6*). They should be avoided in infants, young children, and all patients with dysentery, severe abdominal pain, or high fever (>38°C).

Antimicrobials are not justified in most cases but some complex cases may benefit from specific therapy (*Figure 1*) (see sections *1.4.2 Acute Bacterial Diarrhoea, 1.4.5 Intestinal Parasites, 1.4.6 Traveller's Diarrhoea* and *1.4.7 Antibiotic-Associated Colitis*).

1.4.2

Acute Bacterial Diarrhoea

Acute bacterial diarrhoea may be classified into either *toxigenic*, in which an enterotoxin is the main pathogenic

Notes

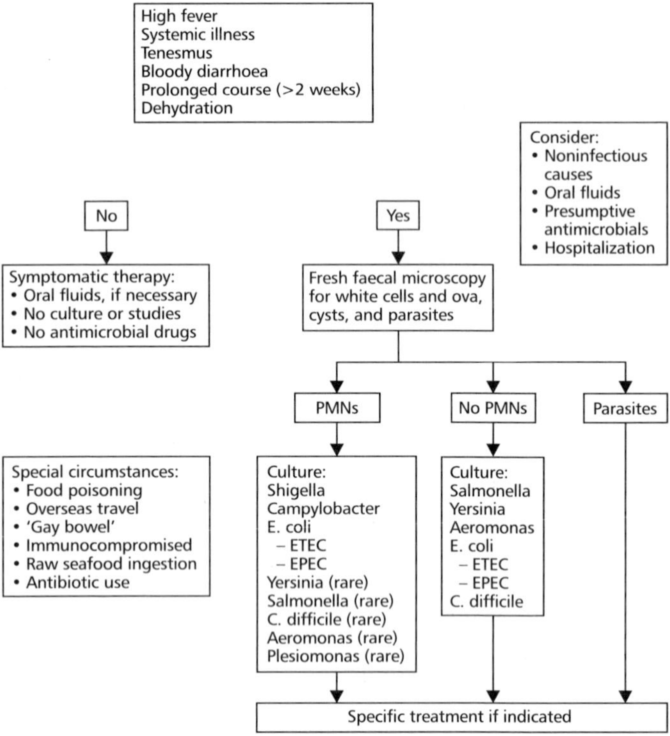

Figure 1 PMNs, polymorphonuclear cells. Adapted from Gorbach SL. Infectious diarrhoea. With permission from Sleisenger MH, Fordtran JS, eds. *Gastrointestinal Disease*. Philadelphia, WB Saunders: 1989.

Notes

mechanism, or *invasive,* in which penetration of the mucosal surface by the organism is the primary event. The toxigenic organisms involve primarily the upper intestine, whereas the invasive pathogens target the lower bowel, especially the terminal ileum and colon. The organisms discussed below produce diarrhoeal illness after colonizing the small or large intestine.

1.4.2.1
TOXIGENIC DIARRHOEA

1.4.2.1.1
Cholera

Cholera is an acute diarrhoeal illness, caused by *Vibrio cholerae* O1, which can cause severe dehydration and death within hours of onset. Faecal fluid output may exceed 20 litres per day, if parenteral fluid replacement is adequate.

EPIDEMIOLOGY AND PATHOGENESIS

V. cholerae O1 is a highly motile Gram-negative, curved, rod-shaped bacterium. There are two main biotypes: *classic* and *El Tor.* The clinical disease is similar with both biotypes, although it tends to be milder with the El Tor vibrio. Cholera is endemic in South-East Asia and has spread in the current pandemic to the Middle East, Africa and southern Europe. There is, however, a very low risk of infection in travellers. The current pandemic began in 1961 and is due to the El Tor biotype.

Notes

V. cholerae O1 is transmitted by contaminated water, food (mainly seafood), and possibly person to person contact. In endemic areas, it is predominantly a disease of children, with prevalence falling with increasing age because of acquired immunity. Individuals with blood group O have greater risk of developing symptomatic disease than those with blood groups A and B, and those with blood group AB have even less risk.

After ingestion of *V. cholerae* O1, the vibrios colonize the proximal small intestine and multiply. The incubation period is usually between 24 and 72 hours. The organism causes no damage to cells, but releases a secretory exotoxin which inhibits sodium absorption and stimulates chloride secretion. There is a net outpouring of isotonic fluid into the small intestinal lumen.

PRESENTATION

It can produce a mild diarrhoeal illness in the majority of symptomatic individuals, or severe diarrhoea. In such cases there is initial vomiting and abdominal distension. Diarrhoea follows with large volumes of "rice-water" stools. Dehydration, acidosis, and hypotension follow rapidly. Stupor, coma, and convulsions (pediatric group) may also be present. Fever is usually absent. Untreated severe cholera has a 30–70% mortality rate.

INVESTIGATIONS

A clinical diagnosis must be made in endemic areas. Similar illnesses may be caused by other organisms, most frequently by enterotoxigenic *Escherichia coli*, but the

Notes

initial treatment is the same. The diagnosis is extremely unlikely if a patient has not recently been in a known endemic or epidemic area.

The organism is usually detectable in fresh stool specimen using dark-field microscopy. White and red cells are absent.

MANAGEMENT

Management involves rapid replacement of fluid and electrolytes. If dehydration is greater than 10%, intravenous rehydration is essential. Most patients can be managed by oral rehydration solutions (ORSs) (see 2.2.2 *Oral Rehydration Solutions*) which contain sodium, potassium, and glucose with either bicarbonate or citrate. The rate of replacement depends on the initial deficit and the rate of continuing losses. About 20 ml kg^{-1} $hour^{-1}$ may be needed for the first few hours, reducing subsequently to about 10 ml kg^{-1} $hour^{-1}$. ORSs have substantially reduced morbidity and mortality.

Several antibiotics decrease the duration and severity of diarrhoea but are not necessary in most cases. Tetracycline 250 mg four times daily (40–50 mg kg^{-1} day^{-1}) for 3–5 days or a single dose of doxycycline (200–300 mg) is commonly effective but resistant strains have been isolated in Bangladesh. *V. cholerae* is also sensitive to ampicillin, chloramphenicol, furazolidone, and co-trimoxazole. Antibiotic administration to home contacts substantially reduces the secondary attack rate.

The current parenterally administered vaccine provides only modest protection in an endemic area, and lasts a few months. Thus it is of use only to travellers and

Notes

should be administered at least 6 days before entering a country that requires vaccination.

1.4.2.1.2

Other vibrios

There are a number of other noncholera vibrios and vibrio-like organisms that cause human diarrhoeal disease, although this is relatively uncommon. These include *V. parahaemolyticus, Aeromonas, Plesiomonas shigelloides, V. cholerae* non-O1, *V. fluvialis, V. vulnificus, V. mimicus, V. hollisae*, and *V. furnissii*. These organisms all like sea water and are associated primarily with molluscs such as crabs, mussels, and oysters. They may produce cytotoxins as well as enterotoxins, and some strains are invasive. Additionally some produce wound infections acquired while swimming.

V. parahemolyticus is an important cause of gastroenteritis in Asia (especially Japan). Infection has also been documented in Australia, Great Britain, and the United States. Diarrhoea, cramps, nausea, and vomiting occur between 3 and 76 hours after ingestion of the organism. Fever and chills may also be present. The duration of illness is usually short (median 3 days). A few patients may experience a dysenteric type illness. Treatment is symptomatic and, although the organism is sensitive to tetracycline or co-trimoxazole, there is no evidence that antibiotics are of any benefit.

Aeromonas infections are usually associated with recent drinking of untreated water. A number of toxins are produced, including an enterotoxin and a cytotoxin.

Notes

Aeromonas may be a common cause of illness, especially in children, ranging from mild to severe diarrhoea. There may be associated blood and mucus. Most cases in children resolve within 1 week. However, in adults chronic diarrhoea is common (mean duration 42 days). It may be possible to shorten a chronic episode with antimicrobials such as tetracycline, co-trimoxazole, or chloramphenicol.

1.4.2.1.3

Escherichia coli

E. coli is a major component of the normal intestinal flora in humans and is usually harmless. There are, however, some that cause diarrhoea by various mechanisms.

Enteropathogenic *E. coli* (EPEC) has been associated with outbreaks of epidemic infantile gastroenteritis. In developed countries these have tended to be in hospitals or nurseries, with newborn or bottle-fed babies at greatest risk. In the tropics, infections are more prevalent in the community with the greatest incidence between the ages of 6 and 18 months – the weaning time. EPEC adheres to the intestinal epithelial cells and produces a toxin, similar to that associated with *Shigella*.

Enterotoxigenic *E. coli* (ETEC) is a major cause of traveller's diarrhoea (see *1.4.6*). ETEC produces toxins that increase fluid secretion in the small intestine.

Enteroinvasive *E. coli* (EIEC) is rare cause of a dysenteric illness similar to that caused by *Shigella*. The organism invades the colonic mucosa and may cause ulceration.

Notes

Enterohaemorrhagic *E. coli* (EHEC) produces a potent cytotoxin and is associated with crampy abdominal pain and bloody diarrhoea with little or no fever.

1.4.2.2 INVASIVE PATHOGENS

1.4.2.2.1 *Shigella*

EPIDEMIOLOGY AND PATHOGENESIS

There are four main subgroups (groups A–D) of *Shigella* consisting respectively of serotypes of *S. dysenteriae, S. flexneri, S. boydi,* and *S. sonnei*. These organisms cause bacillary dysentery which is endemic in tropical and temperate regions. *S. dysenteriae* type 1 (Shiga's bacillus) produces the most severe form of dysentery, and has been responsible for epidemics in Central America, Mexico, and the Indian subcontinent. *S. sonnei* produces the mildest disease. In Britain, Europe and the United States *S. sonnei* accounts for almost all cases. Transmission is essentially from person to person by the faecal–oral route, with simple contamination being sufficient.

Shigella produces a locally invasive colitis by penetration of the colonic wall (and sometimes the terminal ileal wall) to the muscularis mucosae and occasionally may cause a severe necrotizing colitis. In addition, *S. dysenteriae, S. flexneri,* and *S. sonnei* each produce an enterotoxin that is probably the cause of the watery diarrhoea that precedes the dysenteric stage.

Notes

PRESENTATION

The classic clinical features of bacillary dysentery are crampy abdominal pain, rectal burning, fever, malaise, and the frequent passage of bloody mucoid stools. However, this constellation is seen in a minority of infected patients. Many episodes of shigellosis are biphasic with nonbloody watery diarrhoea preceding dysentery of variable severity. The dysenteric component begins 3–5 days after the onset of illness and the volume of stool is usually small. It corresponds to invasion of the colonic mucosa. The colitis may rarely proceed to toxic megacolon.

There is an array of extraintestinal complications associated with bacillary dysentery. These include bacteremia and sepsis, haemolytic uremic syndrome, a leukemoid response, and postinfectious arthritis. In children, meningism is common and seizures may occur.

MANAGEMENT

Mild cases of shigellosis do not require antimicrobial therapy. However, antibiotics are indicated for moderate to severe disease. Ampicillin 500 mg to 1 g orally 6 hourly (children 50–100 $mg\,kg^{-1}\,day^{-1}$ up to the adult dose) for 5–10 days is frequently effective and inexpensive. Amoxycillin is ineffective. Unfortunately, in many countries, plasmid-mediated resistance to ampicillin and other antibiotics is common. Thus, therapy may need to be modified according to culture and sensitivity tests.

Notes

Because shigellosis is very contagious, scrupulous hygiene by people who are in contact with an infected case is very important.

1.4.2.2.2
Salmonella

EPIDEMIOLOGY AND PATHOGENESIS

It is clinically convenient to divide salmonellae into those that cause "enteric fever" (*S. typhi* and *S. paratyphi* A, B, and C, and *S. cholerae-suis,* and rarely other salmonellae), and those that cause acute gastroenteritis such as *S. enteritides* and *S. typhimurium*. Enteric fever is endemic in developing countries with poor sanitation. It is rare in developed countries; in particular the incidence in returning travellers is extremely low. In contrast community-acquired gastroenteritic illness due to salmonellae is an important cause of morbidity and mortality in developed countries but not so in the underdeveloped.

The gastroenteritic group, usually caused by food poisoning, consists of about 2000 potentially pathogenic serotypes. *Salmonella* species are widespread and disease can occur in large outbreaks often associated with a common source, the most common being poultry, meat, eggs, and dairy products.

A number of conditions are associated with an increased risk of salmonellosis. These include the extremes of age, HIV infection, haemolytic anaemia, reduced gastric acid secretion (postsurgical, H_2-antago-

Notes

nist therapy), neoplastic disease (leukemias, lymphomas, disseminated malignancy), and the use of corticosteroids, radiotherapy, and chemotherapy. Schistosomiasis is also associated with recurrent *Salmonella* bacteremia.

Salmonellae infect the ileum and to a lesser extent the colon. They cause mild mucosal ulceration, and spread from the lamina propria to the lymphatics and bloodstream. The extent of mucosal disease is usually less severe than that seen with shigellosis or *Campylobacter* infection. The diarrhoea may be due to both mucosal invasion and the production of a "secretory" factor that stimulates prostaglandin production leading to increased intestinal secretion.

PRESENTATION

There are five clinical syndromes seen with *Salmonella*: (1) gastroenteritis which accounts for about 75% of infections; (2) bacteremia which is detectable in about 10% of cases, and may or may not be associated with gastrointestinal involvement; (3) typhoid or "enteric fever" in 5–10% of infections; (4) localized infections, i.e. osteomyelitis, septic arthritis, endocarditis, pneumonia, meningitis, and focal abscesses, as a result of bacteremia; and (5) chronic asymptomatic carrier state which occurs in less than 1% of infections, with the organism usually being harbored in the gallbladder.

The common gastroenteritic illness has an incubation period of 6–48 hours, depending on the size of the infecting dose. Malaise, nausea, headache, abdominal cramps, and diarrhoea may be preceded by vomiting and fever. The diarrhoea is usually mild and watery, but may

Notes

be severe and either dysenteric or cholera-like in nature. The usual attack lasts 2–3 days, but may be more prolonged with more severe disease.

MANAGEMENT

Simple supportive and symptomatic treatment with oral rehydration fluids is all that is required for most attacks. Antibiotics may shorten the duration of illness, but prolong faecal excretion.

1.4

If diarrhoea is severe or prolonged, or the patient is at "high risk" then ciprofloxacin (500 mg orally every 12 hours for 14 days) is usually suitable. Chloramphenicol 500–750 mg (25 $mg\,kg^{-1}$ up to adult dose) orally 6-hourly for 14 days, or co-trimoxazole 160/800 mg (4/20 $mg\,kg^{-1}$ up to adult dose) orally 12-hourly for 14 days, or amoxycillin 1 g (25 $mg\,kg^{-1}$ up to adult dose) orally 6-hourly for 14 days are also useful. In severe septicemic cases therapy should be started intravenously. Resistance to antibiotics is well recognized.

1.4.2.2.3

Campylobacter

EPIDEMIOLOGY AND PATHOGENESIS

Campylobacter is the most common cause of acute bacterial enteritis. *C. jejuni* is the most frequent species causing diarrhoea. *Campylobacter* species live in cattle, swine, sheep, fowl, and dogs in addition to fresh and salt water. Most human infections probably result from the

Notes

consumption of improperly cooked or contaminated food, especially chicken.

Campylobacter is an invasive pathogen that may involve both small and large intestine. Histologic features include mucosal ulceration, glandular atrophy, mucus depletion, and neutrophilic infiltration with crypt abscess formation.

PRESENTATION

The incubation period is 24–72 hours, although it may extend to 10 days. Diarrhoea and fever are present in 90% of cases, with abdominal pain (70%) and bloody stools (50%). Constitutional symptoms such as headache, malaise, myalgia, anorexia, and vomiting are common. The illness usually lasts about 1 week but relapses may occur in up to a quarter of patients.

MANAGEMENT

Mild cases of *Campylobacter* infection usually do not require antimicrobial therapy. Antibiotics, however, are likely to be helpful when dysentery is present. An effective empiric treatment in adults is ciprofloxacin 500 mg b.i.d. for 5–7 days whilst awaiting culture results. Resistance to fluoroquinolones has been reported. Erythromycin (500 mg (10 $mg\,kg^{-1}$ up to adult dose) q.i.d. for 7 days) is an acceptable alternative and is best for children.

Notes

1.4

1.4.2.2.4
Yersinia

EPIDEMIOLOGY AND PATHOGENESIS

Gastroenteritis due to *Yersinia enterocolitica* can occur worldwide. The organism has been isolated from fresh water and from animals such as cats, chickens, cows, and horses. Animals, as either pets or food sources, are probably responsible for disease transmission.

Yersinia preferentially invades the epithelium overlying intestinal lymphoid tissue, Peyer's patches, and multiplies within lymphoid follicles before spreading to adjacent tissue. The affected gut becomes hyperemic, ulcerated, and infiltrated with neutrophils. Lymphoid hyperplasia (mesenteric adenitis) also occurs.

PRESENTATION

There are several clinical syndromes associated with *Yersinia* that are partly dependent on age. Acute enterocolitis is the most common and occurs most frequently under the age of 5 years, while mesenteric adenitis and terminal ileitis are more common in children over the age of 5 and in adults. The latter syndrome may be mistaken for acute appendicitis. Symptoms can persist for several weeks. In some patients radiographic changes in the terminal ileum resemble Crohn's disease. Seronegative arthropathy or arthritis associated with rash (erythema nodosum and erythema multiforme) are potential long-term sequelae, especially in adults.

Notes

Yersinia bacteremia is uncommon but can lead to metastatic foci in bones, joints, heart, and lungs. Patients at most risk are those with malignancy, diabetes, anaemia, and liver disease.

MANAGEMENT

Y. enterocolitica, a β-lactamase producer, is resistant to penicillin and many cephalosporins. It is susceptible to other antimicrobials (chloramphenicol, aminoglycosides, tetracyclines, co-trimoxazole, "third-generation" cephalosporins, and fluoroquinolones) but there is no evidence that these alter the course of disease.

1.4.3

Bacterial Food Poisoning

Strictly speaking, bacterial food poisoning refers to outbreaks of infection that result from the multiplication of organisms in food.

These may cause large outbreaks as distinct from the odd sporadic case. *Table 14* outlines the main agents that cause foodborne gastroenteritis. Most have been considered elsewhere (see *1.4.2 Acute Bacterial Diarrhoea*). Organisms that will be discussed further in this section are in bold.

Clostridium perfringens

Clostridial food poisoning is usually associated with the ingestion of inadequately cooked meat or poultry which

Notes

1.4

Table 14 Causes of food poisoning

Predominant symptom	Incubation period (hours)	Agent
Diarrhoea	4–12	***Clostridium perfringens***
		Bacillus cereus
	>12	Enterotoxigenic *Escherichia coli*
		Vibrio parahemolyticus
		Cholera
		Other causes of acute diarrhoea
Nausea and vomiting	<2	Heavy metal poisoning
	4–12	***Staphylococcus aureus***
		B. cereus
	>12	Vibrios
		Yersinia enterocolitica
		Other causes of acute vomiting
Nausea, vomiting, and diarrhoea		*Salmonella*
		Campylobacter

has been left to stand for some hours after cooking. The enterotoxin-induced diarrhoeal illness is usually resolved within 12–24 hours and requires no specific treatment. Fatalities are rare.

Staphylococcus aureus

Staphylococcal food poisoning occurs after the ingestion of food contaminated with entertoxin-producing staphylococci. Unrefrigerated, protein-rich foods with a high salt or sugar content are particularly likely to support staphylococci and entertoxin production. The food is

Notes

usually contaminated during preparation. Severe attacks produce vomiting, abdominal pain, and fever. Rarely infection may lead to metabolic alkalosis, hypotension, prostration, and death. In most cases symptoms resolve within 12–24 hours, many before medical attention is sought. The most severe bouts require fluid and electrolyte replacement, and antiemetics. Antibiotics are not appropriate.

Bacillus cereus

There are two clinical types of food poisoning associated with *B. cereus* – a diarrhoeal syndrome and a vomiting syndrome – due to the production of distinct enterotoxins produced by different serotypes. The food is contaminated before cooking. The diarrhoeal syndrome resembles clostridial food poisoning, lasts about 20–36 hours, and is associated with a variety of foods. The vomiting syndrome resembles staphylococcal food poisoning, is usually mild, lasting 8–10 hours, and is usually associated with the consumption of unrefrigerated rice.

1.4.4 Viral Diarrhoea

Acute infective non-bacterial diarrhoea is caused predominantly by viruses. Such infections are a major cause of morbidity and mortality worldwide, especially in infants and children.

Notes

EPIDEMIOLOGY AND PATHOGENESIS

1.4

There are currently four major groups of viruses that are associated with gastroenteritis: rotavirus, enteric adenovirus, calcivirus (including Norwalk and Norwalk-like viruses), and astrovirus. They are spread by faecal–oral means, although airborne spread has been postulated for rotavirus. In temperate climates adenovirus infection occurs throughout the year, whereas rotavirus and astrovirus infection usually occurs in winter. In the tropics rotavirus and astrovirus infection is perennial but may have seasonal variation.

Rotavirus is the main cause of severe gastroenteritis in infants and children. It accounts for up to 70% or more of diarrhoeal illnesses requiring hospitalization in children under 2 years of age. There are often intrafamilial and nosocomial outbreaks. Infants aged less than 3 months of age are relatively resistant because of passive immunity which is acquired transplacentally and from breast milk. The most severe episodes occur between 6 months and 2 years of age. The incubation period is 2–4 days. Rotavirus infects the small intestinal epithelium resulting in enterocyte damage, villus shortening, and crypt hyperplasia. The actual mechanism of diarrhoea, however, is still uncertain. Infection leads to induction of protective antibody-mediated intestinal immunity. Because of persistence of this immunity, infected adults usually do not manifest disease.

Enteric *adenoviruses* are the next most common cause of pediatric gastroenteritis (15–20%). They may also occasionally be pathogens in immunocompromised adults. Most infections occur before 12 months of age, and are

Notes

rare after 2 years. The incubation period is about 8–10 days.

Astrovirus accounts for about 7% of infantile gastroenteritis. It may also be seen in older children up to about the age of 7 years. The incubation period is 3–4 days.

The Norwalk group of *calciviruses* is associated with epidemic gastroenteritis and affects primarily older children and adults. Other calciviruses usually affect infants and young children. Infections can occur throughout the year, but the peak incidence is in winter months. The incubation period is about 1–3 days. Generally the illness lasts 1–2 days. Immunity may only last a few years. Thus people can have repeated infections with specific calciviruses.

PRESENTATION

Viral gastroenteritis is associated with nausea and vomiting as well as diarrhoea; delayed gastric emptying has been demonstrated in children with rotavirus and in adults with calcivirus infection. Most patients are febrile and symptoms may be severe enough to cause clinically significant dehydration. Infections are usually self-limited with resolution within a few days, although in some they may last a couple of weeks. The clinical features cannot be used to distinguish between infecting agents.

Although postinfective small bowel morphologic and physiologic abnormalities usually reverse in 1–2 weeks, secondary lactase deficiency may persist longer.

Notes

INVESTIGATIONS

Major diagnostic tests using faecal specimens include electron microscopy, immune electron microscopy, radio-immunoassay (RIA), enzyme immunoassay (EIA), and reverse transcriptase polymerase chain reaction (PCR). The availability of these tests will vary between laboratories.

Although faecal occult blood and faecal leucocytes are often regarded as markers of invasive bacterial enteritis, they are found frequently in patients with viral diarrhoea.

MANAGEMENT

There is no specific treatment for viral gastroenteritis. The main therapy is supportive with rehydration. In most instances oral fluids, including oral rehydration solutions (see 2.2.2), are sufficient. After a few days there is a gradual return to a normal diet. Restriction of certain carbohydrates, however, may be required temporarily.

Currently vaccines to rotavirus are under development. A number of these are undergoing clinical trial and may be released in the near future.

1.4.5

Intestinal Parasites

Gastrointestinal parasitic infections cause morbidity and mortality worldwide. Underdeveloped countries are primarily affected, but parasitic diseases are increasing in the developed world because of increased foreign

Notes

travel and migration. Parasitic infections are also a problem in patients with HIV infection.

1.4.5.1
PROTOZOAL INFECTIONS

Protozoa survive outside their hosts and ingestion of cysts in food, water, or directly from person to person leads to excystation and the formation of trophozoites which proliferate in the gut. The main protozoal organisms are *Giardia lamblia*, *Entamoeba histolytica*, *Balantidium coli*, *Cryptosporidium*, *Cyclospora*, *Isospora belli*, and microsporidia.

Cryptosporidium, *Cyclospora*, *Isospora belli*, and microsporidia are opportunistic agents. People who are immunosuppressed are the most likely to have significant disease. These protozoa are discussed further in the section on *Diarrhoea in HIV Disease* (see *1.4.8*).

1.4.5.1.1
Giardia lamblia (Giardiasis)

EPIDEMIOLOGY AND PATHOGENESIS

Giardiasis is the most common worldwide protozoal infection of the gastrointestinal tract. It is endemic in developing countries, with young children being most often affected. Symptomatic infection and reinfection are less common in adults, possibly because of "intestinal resistance". In addition to poor sanitation and hygiene,

Notes

risk factors include malnutrition, hypogammaglobulinemia, immunosuppression and possibly reduced acid secretion.

Giardia predominantly colonizes the duodenum and jejunum, and adheres to the epithelial surface. A spectrum of histologic features ranges from normal mucosal microscopy to partial or subtotal villus atrophy. Even in "normal" mucosa there is microvillus damage and functional impairment. The immunologic processes induced by *Giardia* probably contribute to the abnormalities.

Functional derangements are related to the extent of infestation and include impaired absorption of osmotically active solutes and failure of disaccharide hydrolysis leading to a luminal osmotic load. Contributing factors may be reduced pancreatic exocrine function and bile salt uptake by *Giardia*. In some patients bacterial overgrowth may also be present.

PRESENTATION

Giardiasis may present: (1) as asymptomatic cyst excreters (most common in endemic areas); (2) as an acute self-limiting diarrhoeal illness; or (3) as chronic diarrhoea with or without features of malabsorption. The incubation period is about 2 weeks, but may range from several days to 6 weeks.

In the acute form the diarrhoea is watery, yellowish, and offensive, and associated with nausea, anorexia, abdominal bloating, and discomfort. Weight loss is also common. In more than 50% there will be spontaneous improvement in 2–3 weeks. When symptoms persist

---

Notes

diarrhoea can be severe, and about half of these patients will have clinical or biochemical evidence of malabsorption.

INVESTIGATIONS

The diagnosis is often made by the finding of cysts in faecal samples. Excretion is variable and examination of several faecal samples over a period of time may be necessary. Trophozoites may also be seen in direct saline mounts. More recently enzyme-linked immunosorbent assay (ELISA) techniques have become available for the detection of *Giardia* antigens in faeces.

If a diagnosis is not established and giardiasis is still suspected, trophozoites may be found on impression smears of small bowel biopsies or endoscopic brushings. They may also be identifiable on small bowel histology, although they can be hard to see unless specialized stains are used. Examination of small intestinal fluid obtained at endoscopy often identifies trophozoites which may also be retrieved from a fine string carried into the intestine within a gelatin capsule (Entertest).

MANAGEMENT

The nitroimidazoles, metronidazole and tinidazole, are usually effective in giardiasis. Tinidazole 2 g (30–50 $mg\,kg^{-1}$ up to adult dose) orally is given as a single dose. Alternatively, metronidazole can be given as a single oral 2 g (30 $mg\,kg^{-1}$ up to 1.2 g) daily dose for 3 days, or 200–400 mg 8-hourly for 7 (to 14) days, or as a suspension (benzoyl metronidazole) as a single 20–30

Notes

$mg\,kg^{-1}$ (maximum 1.2 g) daily dose for 3 days. Treatment failures do occur on occasion. If persistent infection is confirmed, second-line drugs that may be used are mepacrine and furazolidone.

After treatment there is resolution of diarrhoea over 3–10 days. Other symptoms (i.e. lactose intolerance) may take some months to resolve.

1.4.5.1.2

Entamoeba histolytica (Amoebiasis)

EPIDEMIOLOGY AND PATHOGENESIS

Amebiasis is most prevalent in the developing world, where it is predominantly transmitted by contaminated food and water. In some tropical countries the prevalence exceeds 50%. In many European countries and North America the overall prevalence is 2% or less. However, in the homosexual community of these countries 20–30% are infested but most are asymptomatic carriers who spread the organism sexually.

Ingested cysts develop into trophozoites in the small and large intestine and invade the bowel mucosa, especially the colon. *E. histolytica* is able to penetrate to all layers of the intestinal wall. The resultant inflammation leads to tissue necrosis. The initial small discrete mucosal erosions develop into ulcers which can extend deep into the bowel wall. The intervening mucosa may appear normal. Amebic ulceration is most common in the rectosigmoid region or caecum, but can occur anywhere in the large bowel. Entry of amoebae into the portal

Notes

circulation can lead to hepatic seeding and abscess formation. These frequently extend to adjacent structures.

PRESENTATION

Presenting features range from the asymptomatic carrier to acute dysentery, chronic nondysenteric colonic disease, hepatic abscess, and invasive amebiasis at other sites. Asymptomatic carriage accounts for at least 80–90% of infections.

Acute amebic dysentery is initially mild with nonspecific diarrhoea and mild or moderate abdominal pain. There is subsequent progression to a more severe picture, with dysenteric stools, more severe pain, and tenesmus. Symptoms may stop spontaneously or may wax and wane over a period of weeks or even months. In a few patients the course is more fulminant and may lead to toxic megacolon. Other complications include peritonitis, perforation, and severe haemorrhage.

Mild or right-sided colonic disease may not produce dysenteric symptoms. Alternating diarrhoea and constipation with or without pain, resembling irritable bowel syndrome, are the main features of chronic amebiasis. After an acute or chronic course granulomatous pseudotumours (amebomas) may develop which can mimic carcinoma or Crohn's disease; these are commonest in the caecum and may be multiple. In a few patients healing may also lead to colonic strictures.

Amebic liver abscess is a frequent complication after severe amebic colitis, or may be the primary presentation without previous intestinal symptoms. Fever, sweating,

Notes

and liver pain may be associated with general constitutional upset with weight loss and anaemia. Amebic abscesses may rupture into surrounding tissues including pleura, peritoneum, and pericardium.

INVESTIGATIONS

Invasive intestinal amebiasis is best diagnosed by repeated fresh stool examination for trophozoites using a saline wet-mount preparation. Alternatively, if proctosigmoidoscopic or colonoscopic examination is undertaken, scrapings or biopsies of lesions can be examined but are not foolproof. Cyst detection is best after concentration methods are used.

Serologic tests (i.e. amebic fluorescent antibody test) are most useful for the diagnosis of extraintestinal disease. There are a variety of tests available with sensitivities usually greater than 95% in patients with liver abscess; however, only 60–80% of patients with invasive bowel disease have positive serology. Seropositivity does not distinguish current infection from past disease and may also persist for several years after successful therapy.

MANAGEMENT

The medical therapy for amebiasis is summarized in *Table 15*. Nitroimidazoles are highly effective in intestinal and extraintestinal disease. Metronidazole (pediatric dose 35–50 $mg\,kg^{-1}$ daily in three divided doses) has been used most often. It can be given parenterally in more severe cases. Tinidazole and ornidazole are also

Notes

Table 15 Drug therapy in amebic infections

Type of infection	Drug regimen
Intestinal	
Trophozoites in stool or tissue	**Metronidazole** 600–800 mg orally t.i.d. for 6–10 days *plus or minus* **Diloxanide furoate** 500 mg orally t.i.d. for 10 days (mainly indicated after a short course of metronidazole)
Cyst carriage	**Metronidazole** 600–800 mg orally t.i.d. for 6–10 days *or* **Diloxanide furoate** 500 mg orally t.i.d. for 10 days *or* **Paromomycin sulphate** 500 mg orally t.i.d. for 5–10 days
Extraintestinal	**Metronidazole** 600–800 mg orally t.i.d. for 6–10 days *plus* **Diloxanide furoate** 500 mg orally t.i.d. for 10 days (after metronidazole)

effective. Other effective lumicidal drugs are diloxanide furoate (pediatric dose 20 $mg\,kg^{-1}$ daily in three divided doses) and paromomycin. Drugs such as emetine and dehydroemetine tend not to be used because of the risk of serious side-effects. An exception is the seriously ill patient with threatening toxic megacolon in whom emetine (1 $mg\,kg^{-1}day^{-1}$, maximum 60 mg, by intramuscular or deep subcutaneous injection) may be combined with parenteral metronidazole.

Notes

1.4.5.1.3

Balantidium coli

This human protozoal pathogen is the least common worldwide. It is restricted mainly to tropical and subtropical regions. *B. coli* is carried by pigs, and communities that live in close proximity to these animals are at greatest risk.

PRESENTATION

B. coli produces a colitis that is similar to amebic colitis.

INVESTIGATION

Trophozoites are easily identified in saline wet-mounts of fresh faecal material, in ulcer exudate, or in mucosal biopsy specimens.

MANAGEMENT

Either tetracycline (500 mg orally q.i.d. for 10 days) or metronidazole (800 mg orally t.i.d. for 10 days) is usually effective therapy.

1.4.5.2

INTESTINAL WORM (HELMINTH) INFECTIONS

The helminths discussed below are in intimate contact with the intestinal mucosa in their adult state. Disease associated with them, however, may not primarily be gastrointestinal (i.e. trichinosis).

Notes

EPIDEMIOLOGY AND PATHOGENESIS

Intestinal helminths have a complex lifecycle: some reside in soil and are ingested orally as embryonated eggs that hatch in the upper jejunum (*Ascaris lumbricoides*, whipworm (*Trichuris trichiura*)) or in their larval state penetrate the skin or buccal mucosa (hookworm (*Necator americanus, Ancylostoma duodenale*), *Strongyloides stercoralis*); the infective larvae of schistosomiasis parasites (*Schistosoma mansoni, S. japonicum*) live in fresh water, after release from an intermediate snail host, and penetrate the skin; other helminths are acquired by ingestion of undercooked or raw food infected with worm embryos (*Trichinella spiralis* (main hosts – pigs, boar, bear), beef tapeworm (*Tenia saginata*), pork tapeworm (*Tenia solium*), fish tapeworm (*Diphyllobothrium latum*), *Capillaria philippinensis* (fish)); *Hymenolepis nana* (dwarf tapeworm) is a tapeworm without an intermediate host that is acquired from faecally contaminated food or water; larvae of *Fasciolopsis buski* are acquired from ingestion of raw stems, leaves, and pods of water plants; pinworm (*Enterobius vermicularis*) is spread directly human to human by inhalation and swallowing of eggs.

Helminths that are soil derived and ingested penetrate the bowel wall then return to the lumen to mature (whipworm) or migrate via the liver to lung alveoli (*A. lumbricoides*); those that penetrate the skin gain access to the bloodstream and migrate directly to the lung alveoli; in the lung, larvae may develop into adolescent worms (*S. stercoralis*) before further progression or progress unchanged (hookworms) to the pharynx where they are

Notes

swallowed and mature in the intestines into adult worms, or the immature parasites (*S. mansoni, S. japonicum*) will migrate via the bloodstream to the liver and in the portal venous system develop into adults which migrate to intestinal venules; eggs are released in the intestinal lumen, or in schistosomiasis erode through the gut wall to reach the lumen or transit to the liver. *T. spiralis* (trichinosis) larvae are released in the small intestine; adolescent and adult worms burrow into intestinal tissues and subsequently release larvae; the larvae migrate to muscle and become encysted. Tapeworms, pinworm and *F. buski* have no visceral migration and mature in the intestinal lumen. Adult tapeworms adhere to the luminal surface of the small intestine; they are segmented parasites (each segment is called a proglottid); eggs or gravid proglottids are released and passed in the faeces. Pinworms (*enterobiasis*) are located primarily in the cecal region, and gravid females migrate to the perianal region to deposit their eggs. *F. buski* attach to duodenal and jejunal mucosa and cause deep ulceration at the site of attachment; flukes and ova are passed in the stool or may be vomited.

Helminths are predominantly an infestation that occurs in tropical climates. In endemic areas, infestation is most common in school-age children, especially the malnourished and poverty stricken. Infestations are frequently mixed. *Strongyloides* is most prevalent in the tropics, and may remain a problem throughout life because of autoinfection. Capillariasis occurs mainly in the northern Philippines and Thailand; cases have, however, been described in Egypt and India. *F. buski* is a common parasite in the Orient. The highest incidence

Notes

of *D. latum* is in the Baltic region. Enterobiasis is more common in temperate climates.

PRESENTATION

The gastrointestinal problems associated with helminth infestation are summarized in *Table 16*. Helminth infestations are often asymptomatic or associated with mild chronic symptoms; with moderate to heavy infestations serious problems can occur. There are five helminths that are commonly associated with diarrhoea: *C. philippinensis*, *Schistosoma* (especially *S. mansoni*), *S. stercoralis*, *T. spiralis* (during early phases of infection), and *T. trichiura*. Other helminths that may cause diarrhoea include *H. nana*, *D. latum* and *F. buski*.

S. stercoralis larval hyperinfestation of the colon and perianal region and dissemination throughout the body may occur in the presence of reduced immunity as in malignancy or glucocorticoid therapy.

Helminth migration through the lungs may be associated with fever, cough, and dyspnea due to a pneumonitis (ascariasis, hookworm (occasionally), strongyloidiasis).

INVESTIGATIONS

Initial investigations may be directed at common causes of small or large bowel symptoms, including bacterial and protozoal infections. Determination of HIV status may be appropriate. Peripheral blood eosinophilia, if present, suggests helminthic infestation (especially ascariasis, *F. buski*, strongyloidiasis, trichinosis, and trichuriasis (whipworm)).

Notes

Table 16 Intestinal helminths

Helminth	Adult size	Intestinal sites of adult helminth(s)	Gastrointestine-related problems
Ascariasis (*Ascaris lumbricoides*)	12–35 cm	Small intestine, bile duct	Malnutrition, bowel obstruction or perforation, obstructive jaundice, pancreatitis, appendicitis
Capillariasis (*Capillaria philippinensis*)	2.5–4.3 mm	Small intestinal wall (esp. jejunum)	Borborygmi, watery diarrhoea, steatorrhoea, abdominal pain, weight loss, nausea and vomiting
Hookworm (*Ancylostoma duodenale, Necator americanus*)	15 mm	Duodenum and upper jejunum	Iron deficiency anaemia, protein-losing enteropathy
Flukes (*Fasciolopsis buski* (giant intestinal fluke))	50–75 mm	Duodenum and jejunum	Heavy infections – diarrhoea, protein-losing enteropathy, intestinal obstruction
Pinworm or Threadworm (enterobiasis) (*Enterobius vermicularis*)	2.5–12 mm	Ileum, caecum and proximal colon, perianal region	Pruritus ani, anorexia, weight loss

Table 16 *(continued)*

Helminth	Adult size	Intestinal sites of adult helminth(s)	Gastrointestine-related problems
Schistosomiasis (*Schistosoma japonicum, S. mansoni*)	10–20 mm	Small and large intestinal wall	Chronic bloody diarrhoea
Strongyloidiasis (*Strongyloides stercoralis*)	2–3 mm	Proximal small intestine (stomach to anus)	Abdominal pain, distension, watery diarrhoea (occasionally bloody), urticaria, pruritus ani, malabsorption
Tapeworms (*Diphyllobothrium latum, Hymenolepis nana, Tenia saginata, Tenia solium*)	5–6 m (*H. nana* 25–40 mm)	Small intestine (ileum – *D. latum*)	Nausea, weight loss, pruritus ani (occasionally diarrhoea), megaloblastic anaemia (*D. latum*)
Trichinosis (*Trichinella spiralis*)	1.4–3.2 mm	Small intestinal wall (early phase of infection)	Abdominal pain, nausea and vomiting, diarrhoea
Whipworm (trichuriasis) (*Trichuris trichiura*)	25–50 mm	Large and small intestine	Lower abdominal pain, diarrhoea (occasionally bloody), anaemia

The best method of diagnosis of many helminthic infections is the demonstration of ova or worm segments in the faeces (after concentration techniques for light infections) (ascariasis, capillariasis, *F. buski*, hookworm, schistosomiasis, tapeworms, whipworm), or of larvae in the faeces (strongyloidiasis). Schistosome eggs may also be seen in biopsy specimens, usually rectal. *S. stercoralis* may be cultured from faeces. Strongyloidiasis may also be diagnosed by aspiration of duodenal juice or by the string test (Entertest). Adult worms and/or eggs of *E. vermicularis* can be visualized in the perianal region, usually at night; a strip of sticky tape can be applied to the anal region shortly after waking, and subsequently placed on a microscope slide for visualization.

Upper gastrointestinal endoscopy and small bowel radiology, and colonoscopy or barium enema, may be useful not only in the detection of some helminthic infections, but also in the exclusion of alternative diagnoses – inflammatory bowel disease, colorectal carcinoma, etc.

Serology (ELISA) can detect active infection in schistosomiasis. ELISA may also be useful to detect chronic carriage or recent infection in strongyloidiasis.

MANAGEMENT

Table 17 outlines the main treatment regimens for helminth infections. Mebendazole should not be used in the first trimester of pregnancy or in children under 6 months of age. If a child is under 10 kg, each dose of mebendazole should be reduced to 50 mg.

When *S. stercoralis* hyperinfestation is present, standard therapy may not eradicate the infestation because of

Notes

Table 17 Oral drug therapy in helminth infections

Helminth infection	Drug regimen
Ascariasis	**Piperazine salt** 75 mg kg^{-1} (max. 3.5 g) as a single daily dose for 2 days *or* **Pyrantel embonate** 10–20 mg kg^{-1} (max. 750 mg) as a single dose (do not use if obstruction) *or* **Mebendazole** 100 mg b.i.d. for 3 days
Capillariasis	**Albendazole** 400 mg b.i.d. for 3 days *or* **Mebendazole** 200 mg b.i.d. for at least 20 days
Fluke	**Praziquantel** 25 mg kg^{-1} t.i.d. for 1 day
Hookworm	**Pyrantel embonate** 10–20 mg kg^{-1} (max. 750 mg) as a single dose repeated at 1 week if heavy infection *or* **Mebendazole** 100 mg b.i.d. for 3 days
Pinworm (enterobiasis)	**Pyrantel embonate** 10–20 mg kg^{-1} (max. 750 mg) as a single dose *or* **Mebendazole** 100 mg b.i.d. for 3 days *or* 100 mg as a single dose repeated in 2 weeks
Schistosomiasis	**Praziquantel** 40–50 mg kg^{-1} for 1 day
Strongyloidiasis	**Mebendazole** 100 mg b.i.d. for 3 days *or* **Thiabendazole** 25 mg kg^{-1} (max. 1.5 g) b.i.d. for 3 days *or* **Albendazole** 400 mg b.i.d. for 3 days *or* **Ivermectin** 0.2 mg kg^{-1} daily for 3 days
Tapeworm	**Niclosamide** 2 g as a single dose *or* **Praziquantel** 15–25 mg kg^{-1} as a single dose

Notes

Table 17 (*continued*)

Helminth infection	**Drug regimen**
Trichinosis	**Thiabendazole** 25 mg kg^{-1} (max. 1.5 g) b.i.d. for 5 days Oral **corticosteroids** for severe symptoms during migration and encystation **Mebendazole** 100 mg t.i.d. for 7–14 days for established tissue phase
Whipworm (trichuriasis)	**Mebendazole** 100 mg b.i.d. for 3 days *or* **Albendazole** 400 mg b.i.d. for 1 day

poor absorption and ineffectiveness against larvae in tissues. The worm burden may be minimized, however, by short courses of therapy each month, i.e. thiobendazole 25 mg kg^{-1} b.i.d. for 1 day each month; albendazole 400 mg for 1 day each month; or ivermectin 0.2 mg kg^{-1} for 1 day each month. A similar approach can be used if prolonged immunosuppression is likely in a patient from an endemic area.

In communities with heavy intestinal helminth exposure age-targeted chemotherapy has been shown to improve nutrition, cognitive function and growth. Suitable therapies in such communities are: pyrantel embonate 20 mg kg^{-1} orally (maximum 750 mg), as a single dose every 4 months, or albendazole, 200 mg in patients weighing less than 10 kg or 400 mg in those over 10 kg, as a single dose every 4 months. Once or twice yearly treatment with albendazole (600 mg) has also been demonstrated to be effective.

Notes

1.4.6

Traveller's Diarrhoea

EPIDEMIOLOGY AND PATHOGENESIS

International travel from an industrialized to a developing country is associated with an episode of acute diarrhoea in 20–50% of people. This is usually self-limiting and not harmful. In about 80% of cases the traveller's diarrhoea is associated with an identifiable infectious agent. Causal agents include enterotoxigenic *Escherichia coli* (ETEC) (about 40% of cases); other bacteria (23%), such as *Shigella* species, enteroinvasive *E. coli* (EIEC), *Campylobacter jejuni*, *Salmonella* species, *Aeromonas* species, and *Plesiomonas shigelloides*; viruses (10%), including rotavirus and the Norwalk virus; and protozoa (5%), such as *Giardia lamblia*, *Cryptosporidium parvum*, and *Entamoeba histolytica*. These agents are representative of the environmental or population-carried pathogens of the host country, to which the adult population has developed immunity through childhood infections. The visitor, however, has no such immunity. Consumption of contaminated food and, to a lesser extent, contaminated water are the most important means of acquisition.

PRESENTATION

The symptoms of traveller's diarrhoea often begin within a few days of arriving in a contaminated area. An untreated episode lasts about 2–4 days, but may be briefer. Mild watery diarrhoea with normally coloured stools is the most common presentation (ETEC, *C. parvum*, rotavirus, Norwalk virus, or *C. jejuni*). This may be associated with nausea, vomiting, and abdominal pain. In a few people the acute diarrhoeal episode may progress to malabsorption (*G. lamblia*). In about 20% of cases there will be fever or blood and mucus in the stool (dysentery), or both indicating possible invasive disease (EIEC, *Shigella* species, *Salmonella* species, *E. histolytica*, *C. jejuni*).

MANAGEMENT

Because the illness is usually self-limiting, treatment is supportive and not specifically directed towards the enteropathogen. However, if the diarrhoea persists beyond 7 days or there is more than mild dysentery, stool examination should be undertaken and therapy directed accordingly. The most important aspect of treatment is the replacement of fluid and electrolyte losses with formal oral rehydration solutions, or by high fluid intake of salty soups or fruit juices together with complex carbohydrates such as rice, potato, or bread. In people with watery diarrhoea, *bismuth subsalicylate* (see *2.2.1.2*) reduces stool frequency by about 50%. It also decreases other symptoms associated with viral gastroenteritis. *Loperamide* (see *2.2.1.3*) reduces the frequency of diarrhoea and the duration of illness by up to 80%. Antidiarrhoeal preparations, however, should be avoided in infants, young children, and in all patients with dysentery.

Antibiotic therapy is recommended for diarrhoea associated with moderate to severe abdominal pain,

Notes

fever, or dysentery. Fluoroquinolone antibiotics are the best self-treatment choice for adults travelling to most high-risk places in the world. Examples are ciprofloxacin (500 mg), norfloxacin (400 mg) and ofloxacin (300 mg) taken twice daily for 3–5 days, or even less. Cotrimoxazole (trimethoprim 160 mg and sulphamethoxazole 800 mg), also twice daily as above, is standard therapy for noncoastal areas of Mexico in summer. These antibiotics substantially lessen the duration and severity of illness.

Single-dose antibiotic therapy is effective with mild illness. There is, however, controversy as to whether antibiotics should be used for mild symptoms.

The best preventive measure for traveller's diarrhoea is the avoidance of ingestion of enteropathogens. This is by avoidance of uncooked or unpeeled fruit, ice cubes and tap water, and reheated food left at room temperature. Food should be hotter than 65°C and water boiled or bottled. Unfortunately these measures are difficult to adhere to consistently. Another approach is the selective use of antibiotics (see *Figure 2*). The fluoroquinilones and cotrimoxazole, as above, are effective as single daily doses (reduction in attack rate of more than 80%). They should be commenced on the first day in the at-risk country and continued for 1–2 days after leaving, but should not be taken for more than 3 weeks. These agents have not been recommended routinely because of the small but significant risk of serious adverse effects and concern over the hastening of antibiotic resistance. Bismuth subsalicylate may also reduce the attack rate (by approximately 60%). Other approaches, such as the use of Lactobacillius and vaccines, are under investigation.

Notes

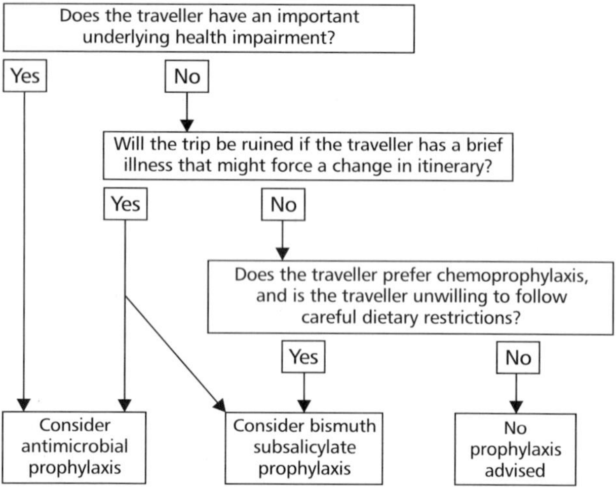

Figure 2 Flow chart for determining the advisability of prophylaxis against traveller's diarrhoea during a stay of less than 3 weeks in a high-risk area of Latin America, Africa, or Southern Asia. With permission from Farthing MJG. Traveller's diarrhoea. *Gut* 1994; **35**: 1–4.

1.4

1.4.7

Antibiotic-associated Colitis and Pseudomembranous Colitis

Antibiotic-associated colitis is inflammation of the colon in association with the recent use of antimicrobials that is otherwise unexplained. Pseudomembranous colitis represents the end of the spectrum of such disease.

Notes

EPIDEMIOLOGY AND PATHOGENESIS

Clostridium difficile, an obligate anaerobic Gram-positive rod, is the major organism implicated in antibiotic-associated colitis and pseudomembranous colitis. Nearly all patients with pseudomembranous colitis have detectable *C. difficile* toxin in the stool. In antibiotic-associated colitis without pseudomembranes the incidence is 50–70%. This decreases to about 10–20% with "simple" diarrhoea. In the latter group the majority of cases have no identifiable cause.

C. difficile releases cytopathic toxins that are detectable in the stool. Antimicrobials alter the normal flora, with reduction in colonization resistance to *C. difficile* which is either a component of the normal flora (approximately 3% of healthy adults) or acquired environmentally. Hospitalized patients receiving antibiotics are at risk of nosocomial infection. The subsequent colitis is toxin mediated. There is no evidence of mucosal invasion by the organism. Although *C. difficile* is often present in infants, adults are far more susceptible to antibiotic-associated colitis. Other potential risk factors are gastrointestinal neoplasia, ischaemia, and surgery.

Nearly all antimicrobials with an antibacterial spectrum of activity have been implicated in pseudomembranous colitis, whereas drugs with a spectrum of activity restricted to mycobacteria, fungi, or parasites appear not to cause this complication. The main drugs have been clindamycin, ampicillin or amoxycillin, and the cephalosporins.

Notes

PRESENTATION

Mild diarrhoea is a common adverse effect of antimicrobial therapy which usually resolves with drug cessation. In some patients, however, the diarrhoea persists or is severe and associated with toxic features such as blood in the stool, fever, and abdominal pain. In a few, the colitis can be severe enough to lead to severe dehydration, electrolyte imbalance, toxic megacolon or colonic perforation, and death.

INVESTIGATIONS

The preferred method to establish the diagnosis of colitis is endoscopy with biopsy and detection of *C. difficile* toxin in the stool. The decision to treat, however, is often based only on clinical symptoms and the presence of toxin.

The distal colon is involved in most patients so that sigmoidoscopic examination is usually adequate. In some, however, the inflammation may be restricted to the right colon, necessitating colonoscopy. In mild disease, there may only be mucosal granularity and friability. With moderate disease there are multiple elevated yellowish-white plaques (pseudomembranes) which vary in size from a few millimetres to 15–20 mm in diameter. The intervening mucosa appears normal or hyperemic and edematous. In more severe disease there is extensive mucosal damage with confluent pseudomembranes.

The histologic appearance ranges from focal necrosis with a polymorphonuclear infiltrate and eosinophilic

Notes

exudate in the lamina propria, with a mushrooming of polymorphs and fibrin from the necrotic focus ("summit lesion"), to glandular disruption, more intense sub-epithelial inflammatory infiltrate, and overlying typical pseudomembranes, to more extensive necrosis with a thick confluent pseudomembrane.

MANAGEMENT

In most patients with antibiotic-associated diarrhoea there is resolution of symptomatology within 1–2 weeks of cessation of the antimicrobial agent.

In persistent or moderate to severe disease supportive measures including intravenous fluids and correction of fluid and electrolyte imbalances may be required. Antiperistaltic drugs should not be given. Systemic corticosteroids may be effective in critically ill patients. Specific treatment may utilize antibiotics directed at *C. difficile* or ion exchange resins to bind the toxin (*Table 18*). In hospital, enteric precautions are recommended to prevent nosocomial spread.

Antibiotic treatment may be with either oral vancomycin, bacitracin, or metronidazole, which are probably therapeutically equivalent. Both vancomycin and bacitracin are poorly absorbed orally and achieve high colonic concentrations without the risk of systemic toxicity. Vancomycin, however, is substantially more expensive. A common problem after treatment is relapse (5–55%), which is comparable between the drugs.

Anion exchange resins bind the toxin. Response to them, however, appears more variable than to the

Notes

Table 18 Specific treatment of *C. difficile* colitis

Antimicrobials	
Oral therapy preferred	
	Vancomycin 125–500 mg orally q.i.d. for 7–14 days
	Bacitracin 500 mg (25 000 units) orally q.i.d. for 7–14 days
	Metronidazole 200–400 mg orally t.i.d. for 7–14 days
Parenteral therapy if oral agents not tolerated	
	Metronidazole 500 mg intravenously 6-hourly
Alternative therapies	
Anion exchange resins	
	Cholestyramine 4-g packet orally t.i.d. for 7–14 days
	Colestipol 5-g packet orally t.i.d. for 7–14 days
Relapses following treatment	
Repeat initial treatment followed by	
	Cholestyramine 4-g packet orally t.i.d. for 2–3 weeks or *vancomycin* 125 mg orally on alternate days for 2–3 weeks

antimicrobials. Thus they are generally reserved for the less seriously ill patient. Cholestyramine should not be administered with vancomycin because it binds the antibiotic and reduces colonic levels. Other analogueous reactions have not been examined.

Relapses may occur 3–10 days after therapy is discontinued. The organism remains sensitive to the antimicrobials. Most will improve without specific therapy. However, if clinically necessary, the initial therapy could be repeated followed by a more prolonged course of cholestyramine or vancomycin. Alternative approaches to re-establishing the normal colonic flora using lactobacilli or faecal enemas have not been studied adequately.

Notes

1.4.8

Diarrhoea in HIV Disease

Diarrhoea occurs in 50–90% of patients during the course of HIV disease. It may be either acute or chronic (three or more liquid motions daily for more than 1 month in HIV-infected patients), and can be severely incapacitating and difficult to treat. A wide variety of bacterial, protozoal, and viral pathogens has been implicated in HIV-associated diarrhoea.

EPIDEMIOLOGY AND PATHOGENESIS

Infection with HIV results in a progressive loss of T helper (CD4) cells which precedes the development of symptoms and predicts the clinical course. Additionally there are functional lymphocyte abnormalities including impaired cytotoxicity and reduced antibody-mediated immune function. These changes may particularly affect mucocutaneous immunity. There are also nonspecific alterations of host resistance, such as reduced gastric acid secretion, in some HIV-infected individuals.

Diarrhoea in patients with HIV infection and CD4 cell counts greater than 200 per mm^3 is most likely to be due to nonopportunistic pathogens such as *Salmonella, Campylobacter,* and *Shigella*. These pathogens are usually foodborne but can be transmitted sexually. Other pathogens that are common and are more likely related to sexual activity include *Neisseria gonorrhoea, Treponema pallidum,* and *Chlamydia trachomatis,* which may cause proctitis with mild diarrhoea; *Giardia* infection may produce a watery diarrhoea or steatorrhoea.

Notes

In patients with CD4 counts lower than 200 per mm^3 there is an increased likelihood of opportunistic infections including parasites (*Cryptosporidium, Cyclospora,* microsporidia (*Enterocytozoon bineusi* or *Septada intestinalis*), and *Isospora belli,* viruses (cytomegalovirus (CMV), adenovirus, and herpes simplex virus) and bacteria (*Mycobacterium avium intracellulare* (MAI)). Infections with nonopportunistic pathogens (*Salmonella, Campylobacter,* and *Shigella*) are also more likely to be associated with bacteremia and increased relapse.

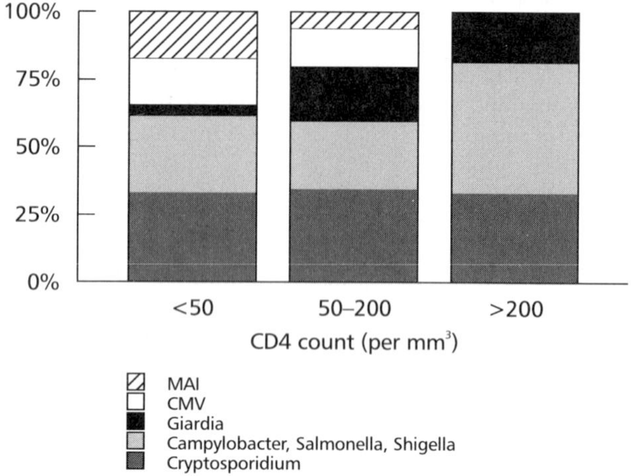

Figure 3 Identifiable infective causes of chronic diarrhoea in patients with different CD4 counts. Adapted from Gazzard B and Blanshard. AIDS and other immunodeficiency states. *Baillière's Clinical Gastroenterology* 1993; 1: **387–419** (with permission).

Notes

In 20–40% of HIV-positive patients with chronic wasting diarrhoea a pathogen will not be identifiable. In some, small bowel lymphoma or Kaposi's sarcoma may be the cause. The remainder are regarded as having an AIDS enteropathy. This may be related directly to HIV infection or to as yet unrecognized enteric pathogens.

PRESENTATION

The clinical history can be useful in localizing the level of the gastrointestinal tract involved and in delineating potential pathogens. Recent travel exposes the individual to a variety of pathogens (see *1.4.6 Traveller's Diarrhoea*) with the risk of persistent illness if immunosuppression is present. If there has been dietary indiscretion with raw shellfish, consider viruses and noncholera vibrios; with unpasteurized dairy products consider *Salmonella, Campylobacter,* and *Cryptosporidium;* with undercooked pork consider *Yersinia.* Recent antibiotic use raises the possibility of *Clostridium difficile* (see *1.4.7*). Drugs used in patients with HIV infection such as zidovudine and didanosine can cause diarrhoea. Sexual promiscuity broadens the differential diagnosis to include organisms that may be transmitted sexually.

Symptoms of cramps, bloating, and nausea suggest gastric or small bowel involvement (*Cryptosporidium, Giardia,* microsporidia or *Isospora belli*); blood in the motions implies colonic involvement (CMV, *Shigella,* or *Campylobacter*); tenesmus may be due to herpes, *Shigella,* or *Campylobacter.*

Notes

INVESTIGATIONS

Tests should identify treatable diseases but minimize diagnostic invasiveness. In patients with CD4 counts above 200 per mm^3 stool culture and microscopy should suffice; for those with lower CD4 counts more extensive investigations are usually needed. Stool culture is undertaken, but stools should also be examined for *Cryptosporidium*, microsporidia, other parasites, and helminths. If the CD4 count is lower than 150 per mm^3, stools are also cultured for MAI. They are unlikely to be positive in less immunocompromised patients. Repeated sampling may be necessary for cryptosporidiosis as some patients who shed the organism only intermittently. Frequently, coinfection by more than one enteric pathogen complicates evaluation.

If symptoms are colonic in nature, flexible sigmoidoscopy may be appropriate with biopsy for histopathology, especially for CMV and herpesvirus. In diarrhoea that might originate from the small bowel, jejunal biopsy or duodenal aspiration can have a reasonable diagnostic yield. Jejunal biopsy may show histologic evidence of cryptosporidial, giardial or *Isospora* infection, and may be the main method available for diagnosis of microsporidiosis. Serology is of little use in CMV disease and the diagnosis is dependent on the finding of CMV inclusions in biopsy specimens.

MANAGEMENT

If enteric pathogens for which there are specific therapies are found then treatment should be administered. Bacterial diarrhoea may require prolonged antibiotic

Notes

therapy (weeks to months) to prevent recurrence. *Giardia* infection is treated with standard therapy (see *1.4.5.1.1*). Sometimes diagnosis may be difficult, in which case empiric treatment is warranted.

The most common opportunistic infection, with *Cryptosporidium parvum*, is one of the least responsive to therapy. A variety of macrolide antibiotics (erythromycin, spiramycin, azithromycin) have been tried. Possibly the most effective in reducing stool volume is paromomycin, but cryptosporidia are rarely eradicated.

There is no consistently effective treatment for microsporidia. Metronidazole may transiently improve symptoms but does not eradicate the organism. Some patients may also respond to albendazole (400 mg twice a day). Those infected with *Septada intestinalis*, however, appear to be more responsive and may actually clear the organism. *Isospora belli* infection is responsive to trimethoprim sulphamethoxazole. Maintenance therapy is recommended because recurrence is common. Alternatives include pyrimethamine and diclazuril.

Ganciclovir (5 $mg\,kg^{-1}$ i.v., 12 hourly, for 2 weeks) is effective in most patients with CMV disease. If ganciclovir is contraindicated or ineffective then foscarnet (180 $mg\,kg^{-1}\,day^{-1}$, either continuously or in three divided doses, for 2 weeks) is often an effective alternative.

There is no clearly effective therapy for MAI. Regimens with four or five antimicrobial agents – including isoniazid, rifabutin, clofazimine, cycloserine, ciprofloxacin, amikacin, imipenem, ethambutol, and others – have been tried, some with partial improvement in symptoms. Recently azithromycin and clarithromycin have been demonstrated to have possible benefit.

Notes

Specialist advice should be sought before therapeutic intervention.

When no pathogen has been identified or in unresponsive opportunistic infections the mainstay of treatment is symptomatic with opiates (see *2.2.1.3 Opioids*) for diarrhoea and oral rehydration solutions (see *2.2.2*). Synthetic somatostatin analogueues have had benefit in some patients, although relapse tends to occur despite continuing therapy.

1.4.9

Overview of Malabsorption

Malabsorption is a term that encompasses the impairment of normal digestion or absorption, which may be caused by a multitude of diseases (*Table 19*). These diseases can result in either limited or extensive nutritional deficiency. The clinical manifestations are also diverse and dependent on the area of the gastrointestinal tract involved and the degree of functional impairment.

This section outlines the presentation, investigation, and therapy of malabsorption in general. Specific diseases are addressed subsequently in this book.

PRESENTATION

The clinical features are given in *Table 20*. While many symptoms are nonspecific, a careful history provides clues to etiology. Many of the diseases associated with malabsorption have specific features which may give further clue to the diagnosis.

Notes

Table 19 A classification of malabsorption

Mucosal defect

Structural

Coeliac disease (gluten enteropathy)
Tropical sprue
Whipple's disease
Lymphangiectasia

Functional

Disaccharidase deficiency (lactase deficiency)
Select deficiency of amino acid, folate, and vitamin B_{12} transport
Abetalipoproteinemia

Structural defect

Crohn's disease
Short bowel
Fistulae, blind loops, diverticula, strictures
Radiation enteritis
Intestinal ischaemia
Amyloidosis
Eosinophilic gastroenteropathy
Small intestinal lymphoma
Gastric resection: rapid gastric emptying, intestinal hurry, afferent loop pooling and bacterial overgrowth, reduced stimuli to biliary and pancreatic secretions, pancreatic atrophy

Infective

Infective diarrhoea (including diarrhoea in HIV disease)
Bacterial overgrowth
Anatomic: blind loops, diverticula, strictures, pseudo-obstruction
Abnormal motility: diabetes mellitus, scleroderma

Notes

Table 19 (*continued*)

Maldigestion

Pancreatic enzyme deficiency or inactivation

Chronic pancreatitis

Cystic fibrosis

Pancreatic carcinoma

Pancreatic resection

Zollinger–Ellison syndrome

Bile salt deficiency

Severe parenchymal liver disease

Cholestatic liver disease

Bile duct obstruction

Drugs (see *Section B*)

Antacids, anticonvulsants, cholestyramine, clindamycin, colchicine, ethanol, metformin, methotrexate, neomycin, para-aminosalicylic acid, paraffin oil, phenindione, sulphasalazine, tetracycline

Lymphatic obstruction

Primary intestinal lymphangiectasia, intestinal lymphoma, cardiac disease, metastatic carcinoma or mesothelioma, retroperitoneal fibrosis, tuberculosis

Extraintestinal disease

Adrenal insufficiency, diabetes mellitus, hyperthyroidism, hypoparathyroidism, hypogammaglobulinemia, carcinoid syndrome

(This is not a full coverage of conditions that may be associated with malabsorption. Conditions mentioned may cause malabsorption by more than one mechanism. Conditions that are discussed further are italicized.)

Notes

Table 20 Clinical features and pathophysiology in malabsorption

System	Clinical feature	Pathophysiology
Gastrointestinal	Diarrhoea	Decreased absorption and increased secretion of water and electrolytes; impaired fatty acid and bile salt absorption
	Steatorrhoea	Impaired fatty acid and bile salt absorption
	Weight loss with hyperphagia	Malabsorption of carbohydrate, fat, and protein with inadequate calorie replacement
	Flatus, borborygmus, distension	Bacterial fermentation of unabsorbed carbohydrate
	Abdominal pain	Small intestinal stricture, pancreatic infiltration, intestinal ischaemia
	Glossitis, cheilosis, stomatitis	Decreased vitamin B_{12}, folate, and iron absorption
Genitourinary	Nocturia	Delayed water absorption, hypokalemia
	Renal impairment	Fluid and electrolyte depletion
	Amenorrhoea	Calorie and protein deficiency
Haematopoietic	Anaemia	Decreased vitamin B_{12}, folate, and iron absorption
	Easy bruising, petechiae, haematuria	Decreased vitamin K absorption

Table 20 *(continued)*

System	Clinical feature	Pathophysiology
Musculoskeletal	Muscle wasting, oedema	Decreased protein absorption or loss
	Muscle cramps, weakness	Hypokalemia
	Tetany, paresthesiae	Vitamin D deficiency, hypocalcemia, hypomagnesemia
	Bone pain	Protein depletion, vitamin D deficiency, hypocalcemia
Nervous	Night blindness, xerophthalmia	Vitamin A deficiency
	Peripheral neuropathy	Vitamin B_{12} and thiamine deficiency
Skin	Hyperkeratosis	Vitamin A deficiency
	Acrodermatitis	Zinc deficiency

INVESTIGATIONS

Initial investigations include estimation of electrolytes (including calcium, magnesium, and zinc), urea and liver function tests, fasting glucose, thyroid function tests, fasting cholesterol and triglycerides, haematology (including iron studies, red cell folate, and vitamin B_{12} levels), and prothrombin time. The clinical history and features, and the results of initial investigation, usually direct further investigation.

The following tests may be used to document malabsorption.

Faecal fat. Fat absorption can usually be estimated by measuring faecal fat excretion. Normal faecal fat excretion measured over 5 days, on a diet of 70–100 g fat per day, is 7 g or less per day. Proportionally higher excretion of faecal fat occurs when dietary fat is increased. Thus it is important to know the dietary fat intake before interpreting any result. Faecal fat can be expressed as a percentage of dietary fat, with 7% representing the upper limit of normal. Because of irregularity of bowel habit, collection should be for at least 5 days. Faecal markers or stool softeners may improve the accuracy of the collection. Many laboratories refuse to analyse faecal collections.

Other tests of fat malabsorption include macroscopic and microscopic examination of faeces (not useful in mild steatorrhoea); estimation of serum carotene (low concentrations may also be present with poor dietary intake and with liver disease); and the use of radioactive fats, such as the ^{14}C-triolein breath test (which is not as sensitive or specific as direct measurement).

Notes

Carbohydrate absorption. The measurement of breath hydrogen after oral intake of a standardized amount for carbohydrate is a simple investigation of carbohydrate malabsorption. Carbohydrates commonly used include fructose, glucose, lactose, lactulose, and sucrose. Non-absorbed carbohydrate is fermented by bacteria, in the colon or in regions of bacterial overgrowth, with production of hydrogen which appears rapidly in the breath. The hydrogen breath test is most commonly used to diagnose *lactase deficiency.*

An alternative is the assay of disaccharidase activity in small bowel biopsy specimens.

Carbohydrate absorptive capacity can also be tested using D-xylose. Xylose is a pentose which is incompletely absorbed in the small intestine by the same transport mechanisms as glucose and galactose. After absorption the majority is excreted unchanged in the urine. A normal person will excrete at least 2 g of a 5-g oral dose of xylose in 5 hours. If steatorrhoea is present, a D-xylose absorption test is useful in differentiating between small intestinal mucosal disease (reduced excretion) and pancreatic insufficiency (normal excretion). Bacterial overgrowth will also reduce xylose excretion, but this is likely to be increased after oral antibiotics. Xylose excretion may also be reduced by renal impairment and ascites.

Protein absorption. In many disorders of the gastro-intestinal tract there is excessive luminal loss of protein. This loss can exceed the synthetic capacity of the liver and hypoalbuminemia develops. Radiolabelled proteins can be given intravenously to examine plasma protein kinetics (^{131}I-albumin, ^{131}I-gammaglobulin) or enteric loss

Notes

(^{51}Cr-albumin, ^{51}Cr-chloride (labels proteins after injection)). A nonisotopic method is to measure the faecal clearance of α_1-antitrypsin which is normally resistant to hydrolysis, and its clearance correlates well with ^{51}Cr clearance. However, α_1-antitrypsin is degraded by gastric acid and is therefore not a useful measure if protein loss is gastric.

Demonstration of malabsorption does not provide a definitive diagnosis, which for many diseases comes from a small bowel biopsy obtained endoscopically or by Crosby capsule. The material obtained can be used for histopathology, cytology, culture, and enzyme analysis. Other investigations that may help to provide a specific diagnosis include small bowel radiology, pancreatic function tests, and tests for bacterial overgrowth.

MANAGEMENT

Dietary supplementation is an important part of the general management of a patient with malabsorption. This should be directed towards correcting specific deficiencies (*Table 21*). Antidiarrhoeals may be helpful (see *2.2.1 Antidiarrhoeals*) or cholestyramine (4-g sachet before meals), for bile salt overflow. Specific therapy for many of the diseases associated with malabsorption are discussed further in the relevant sections of this book.

1.4.10

Coeliac Disease

Coeliac disease is the commonest and most important cause of malabsorption in the developed world. It is

Notes

Table 21 Dietary supplements*

	RDI	Supplementation
Calcium	800 mg	Oral: calcium carbonate tablets or capsules 350–1500 mg, 1–2 daily with food; calcium gluconate tablets 600 mg to 1 g, 1–2 daily; calcium lactate tablets 350–1500 mg, 1–2 daily Intravenous: calcium gluconate 10%, 10–30 ml slowly
Folate	200 mg	Oral: folic acid tablets 0.5–5 mg, 1 daily with food
Fat-soluble vitamins		
A	2250–4000 IU	Oral: vitamin A capsules (3–15 mg retinol, 10 000–50 000 IU), 2 daily for 3 days, then 1 daily for 2 weeks Deep intramuscular: vitamin A 50 000 IU per ml; deficiency – 2 ml monthly, increased to weekly in acute deficiency; courses no longer than 6 weeks with a 2-week interval
D	5–10 mg	Oral: ergocalciferol (D_2) 250 mg tablets, up to 1 mg (100 000 IU) daily; increase dose as necessary to maintain normal serum calcium level
E	8–10 mg	Oral: D-α-tocopherol 100–500 IU, 1–2 daily with food
K	60 mg	Oral: menadiol 10 mg tablet, 1 daily; phytomenadione 10 mg tablet, 1 daily Intravenous: phytomenadione 2 mg ml^{-1}, 10 mg daily

Table 21 (*continued*)

	RDI	Supplementation
Iron	800 mg	Oral: ferrous sulphate 150–325 mg, three times daily Deep intramuscular: iron dextran (Imferon) 50 mg ml^{-1} of iron, initial 0.5-ml test dose, up to 5 ml at a time (half dose in each buttock), because of slow-release; adjust frequency according to anaemia
Magnesium	Females 280 mg Males 350 mg	Oral: magnesium gluconate tablet 500 mg, 1–4 g daily Intramuscular: magnesium sulphate 50% solution, 2 ml 2–3 times daily
Vitamin B_{12}	2 mg	Intramuscular: hydroxocobalamin 1 mg ml^{-1}, initially 1 mg repeated 5 times over 2 weeks, maintenance 1 mg every 3 months; cyanocobalamin 1 mg ml^{-1}, initially 1 mg repeated 10 times over 4 weeks, maintenance 1 mg every month
Zinc	12–15 mg	Oral: zinc sulphate tablets or capsules 22–220 mg, 1–3 daily with food

** If severe deficiency, replacement may need to be intravenous and in larger amounts. RDI, recommended daily intake.*

defined as an abnormal small intestinal mucosa that improves morphologically when treated with a gluten-free diet and that deteriorates again on the reintroduction of gluten.

EPIDEMIOLOGY AND PATHOGENESIS

The prevalence of coeliac disease varies considerably in different parts of the world. It is highest in Galway, Ireland (1 in 300 population) and up to 1 in 3000 in other parts of Europe. It is rare in noncaucasians. The clinical expression of coeliac disease requires the interaction of environmental genetic factors. The main environmental factor is gliadin which is derived from gluten, the water-insoluble protein fraction of cereal grains. Over 90% of caucasians with coeliac disease have the HLA-DR3 and HLA-DQ2 haplotype. However, there is only 70% concordance in monozygotic twins and it is clear that other environmental factors are important in the pathogenesis of the disease. It has been suggested that infection with adenovirus type 12 is the additional factor needed which causes cross-reactivity with gluten. However, it is still unclear as to how gluten damages the mucosa, although it is recognized that sensitized T cells mediate the epithelial damage.

PRESENTATION

The disease may present any time from the first months of life to the eighth decade. In childhood the clinical features are usually failure to thrive, abdominal distension, steatorrhoea, and anorexia. In contrast, adult coeliac

Notes

disease may present in a variety of ways. The most common presenting features are diarrhoea, weight loss, and anaemia, although other presentations include aphthous ulceration, skin rashes, and abdominal discomfort. The clinical findings are shown in *Table* 22. Coeliac disease is associated with a number of other diseases including diabetes mellitus, fibrosing alveolitis, and dermatitis herpetiformis.

INVESTIGATIONS

Haematological investigations may indicate an anaemia which may be an iron, folate, or mixed dimorphic picture due to a combination. Vitamin B_{12} deficiency is rarer and indicates involvement of the ileum. Hyposplenism which occurs in approximately 30% of coeliacs, may produce an abnormal blood film with Howell–Jolly bodies present. Serologic testing reveals antigliadin antibodies in only about 60% of patients but the endomysial antibody is more specific and sensitive, being found in about 80% of adult coeliac patients. This antibody has the advantage of

Table 22 Clinical physical findings in coeliac disease

Common	Uncommon
Weight loss	Clubbing
Angular stomatitis	Ascites
Glossitis	Neuropathy
Abdominal distension	Ataxia
Aphthous ulceration	Tetany
	Pigmentation
	Muscle wasting

Notes

disappearing after successful withdrawal of gluten. The endomysial antibody is usually an immunoglobulin (Ig) A antibody and can be negative in patients who have IgA deficiency, which is found in about 2% of coeliac patients.

The gold standard of diagnosis is a small intestinal biopsy, either from the duodenum at endoscopy or from the jejunum by means of a suction capsule biopsy, showing partial or total villous atrophy.

MANAGEMENT

The treatment of coeliac disease consists of complete withdrawal of gluten from the diet. In practice, this means a total avoidance of wheat, rye, and barley. Approximately 15% of adult patients will not respond to gluten withdrawal and in these patients *prednisolone* is the best treatment. The initial dose is 40–60 mg daily, reducing to the minimal dose needed to maintain remission. Prednisolone is usually continued indefinitely and *azathioprine* should be considered as a steroid-sparing agent in patients who require long-term high-dose prednisolone. Rarely, concurrent pancreatic exocrine failure can occur and should be considered in patients in whom jejunal histology improves but steatorrhoea persists. Malnourished patients may require supplementation with vitamins and minerals.

Patients need to adhere to gluten withdrawal for life and it is believed that this reduces the chance of developing complications such as intestinal T-cell lymphoma. In addition, adenocarcinoma has been found to occur in increased prevalence in coeliac disease and the overall mortality rate of coeliac patients is twice that of the general population.

Notes

1.4.11

Tropical Sprue

Tropical sprue is a chronic malabsorption disorder acquired by indigenous people or visitors (usually for greater than 6 months' duration) in endemic tropical areas. It is characterized by abnormalities of small bowel structure and function which lead to the development of nutritional deficiencies, and which respond to treatment with folic acid and tetracycline.

EPIDEMIOLOGY AND PATHOGENESIS

Tropical sprue is endemic in the West Indies, especially Puerto Rico, Cuba, the Dominican Republic and Haiti; the northern part of South America; India and South-East Asia. It has also been found in the native populations of Nigeria, Zimbabwe, and South Africa. The incidence of the disorder is difficult to assess because of lack of the necessary diagnostic tests.

Tropical sprue, although usually sporadic in occurrence, may at times be epidemic as a sequela of outbreaks of acute diarrhoeal disease. Adults are affected more commonly than children. It tends not to develop in the rainy season. It can develop in expatriates within a few weeks of arrival in an endemic area, but usually they have been resident for 2 years or more. Occasionally, overt symptoms may not be obvious for months or years after leaving an endemic area.

Tropical sprue is probably an infectious disease caused by chronic intestinal contamination with one or more enteric pathogens. This is suggested by its characteristics of spread in epidemics with clustering in time and space,

Notes

and response to antibiotics. As the disorder can occur in well-nourished individuals, it is unlikely that dietary factors are causative. Although a gluten-free diet may result in some histologic and clinical improvement, tropical sprue can occur in populations that do not consume gluten.

Small intestinal morphologic abnormalities are a characteristic feature. Under the dissecting microscope, villi appear thickened and coalesced to form leaves, ridges, and convolutions; the flat biopsy, as seen in coeliac disease, is rare. On histology the mucosa shows partial villous atrophy with elongated crypts, shortened broad villi, and chronic inflammatory cell infiltration of the lamina propria. Changes may be milder earlier in the course of the disease. Initially the upper small intestine is affected, but later changes involve the ileum as well. Additionally, gastric histology may demonstrate superficial or complete atrophic gastritis, which may be associated with reduced gastric acid and intrinsic factor secretion.

An additional histologic feature is an abnormal pattern of lipid accumulation in small intestinal mucosa which is characteristic, but not pathognomonic, of tropical sprue. Lipid staining demonstrates the accumulation of lipid droplets located mainly subjacent to the surface epithelium. In contrast, in coeliac disease the lipid is within the surface epithelium; in normal biopsies it is present in the basal portions of the lamina propria.

PRESENTATION

The clinical features at presentation are varied and relate to the duration of disease. Initially there is chronic, mild,

Notes

non-bloody diarrhoea which may be associated with abdominal cramps and distension, fever, malaise, and fatigue. As the disease progresses more characteristic features of malabsorption develop (see *1.4.9 Overview of Malabsorption*). Of particular note is folate and vitamin B_{12} deficiency. In about 10% of patients, nutritional deficiencies may develop in the absence of diarrhoea.

INVESTIGATIONS

Enteric bacterial pathogens and parasites require exclusion (see *1.4.1 Overview of Infectious Diarrhoea*). On initial investigation, megaloblastic anaemia, due to combined folate and vitamin B_{12} deficiency, is usually present in advanced tropical sprue. The vitamin B_{12} malabsorption is not corrected by the addition of intrinsic factor. Other tests may demonstrate abnormalities of carbohydrate, fat, and protein malabsorption (see *1.4.9 Overview of Malabsorption*). Radiology is done to exclude other disorders. Small bowel biopsy (see above) is the most useful diagnostic investigation. Final confirmation of diagnosis, however, rests with response to treatment.

MANAGEMENT

Treatment consists of correction of deficiencies (see *1.4.9*), especially folate and vitamin B_{12} deficiency, and antibiotics. The antimicrobials presumably eradicate the organisms responsible for the disease. The most effective are tetracycline and poorly absorbed sulphonamides. Appropriate therapy is tetracycline 1 g daily for 1 month, then 500 mg per day for 5 months or until evidence is

Notes

obtained that intestinal function has returned to normal. Folate (5 mg per day) is usually also given for a prolonged period of time. Successful treatment results in restoration of normal intestinal morphology.

1.4.12

α Chain Disease (Mediterranean Lymphoma)

This condition occurs over much of the tropics, but is particularly common around the Mediterranean, Middle East, South-East Asia, and southern Africa. It consists of a diffuse lymphoplasmacytic proliferation associated with α heavy chains in the serum and other biologic fluids.

EPIDEMIOLOGY AND PATHOGENESIS

The etiology is unknown. It has been suggested that chronic infections and possibly genetic factors are important. The disease usually involves the upper jejunum. It affects young adults and children, particularly of low socioeconomic groups and there is an equal sex incidence.

PRESENTATION

Patients present with chronic diarrhoea, abdominal pain, and some severe chronic malabsorption, and later in the disease small intestinal obstruction.

Notes

INVESTIGATIONS

α chains can be detected by immunoelectrophoresis in a serum sample; hypoalbuminemia and a raised serum alkaline phosphatase concentration are common. Small intestinal biopsy shows lymphocytic proliferation which is usually in the lamina propria. Villons atrophy is often present. Initially, mesenteric lymph gland involvement is seen, but later in the disease there is involvement of the major abdominal organs with multicentric tumour masses being present.

MANAGEMENT

When commenced early, tetracycline often produces a remission in the lymphoplasmacytic proliferation. In later cases cytotoxic agents such as cyclophosphamide often accompanied by *prednisolone* are used. The progress of the condition depends on the extent of the disease involvement at presentation.

1.4.13

Whipple's Disease

Whipple's disease is a rare systemic disorder which is important to recognize because appropriate treatment can provide a cure, and prevent what would have been an inexorable progression to death.

Notes

EPIDEMIOLOGY AND PATHOGENESIS

Although Whipple's disease can occur at any age, it is most common in the fourth and fifth decades of life. Males are affected more than females (approximately 10:1) with most being caucasian.

Whipple's disease may affect many organs; however, the histopathologic features of the small intestinal mucosa are often the key to the diagnosis. The main diagnostic feature is infiltration of the lamina propria by foamy macrophages which contain multiple large granules which stain with periodic acid–Schiff (PAS). These granules are lysosomes with the endproducts of bacterial digestion. High-resolution light microscopy or electron microscopy reveals multiple tiny bacilli (1–2.5 μm long and 0.25 μm wide) in the epithelium, lamina propria, submucosa, and macrophages. The bacilli have been isolated from involved tissue and are claimed to be an aerobic *Corynebacterium*, a *Haemophilus* species, a *Brucella*-like organism, or a streptococcus. Treatment with appropriate antibiotics leads to gradual reversion of the mucosa towards normal. In some cases the small intestinal mucosa is not involved or relapse occurs without intestinal involvement.

The PAS-positive macrophages may also be identified in other organs including heart, lung, liver, spleen, kidneys, large intestine, central nervous system, and lymph nodes.

PRESENTATION

Extraintestinal symptoms may precede overt gastrointestinal features by many years. Arthritis and fever

Notes

are the most common. Polyarthralgia or polyarthritis of variable severity is present in about two thirds of patients. Significant fever, usually mild, is present in more than half the cases. Cough and pleuritic pain are quite common. Occasionally pulmonary involvement can mimic sarcoidosis. Cardiac disease can result in congestive heart failure, pericarditis, and endocarditis. Neurologic symptoms (in less than 10% of cases) include dementia, headache, convulsions, psychosis, and central motor, sensory, and coordination deficits.

Gastrointestinal symptoms are initially nonspecific and include anorexia, occasional abdominal pain, and diarrhoea. The diarrhoea, as it progresses, becomes that of frequent steatorrhoeal stools associated with weight loss and other features of severe malabsorption.

Many of the clinical features are those associated with malabsorption (see *1.4.9 Overview of Malabsorption*). Additionally moderate peripheral lymphadenopathy is common. There are also signs that reflect other organ involvement.

INVESTIGATIONS

Small bowel biopsy, as noted above, is the most important investigation. Otherwise abnormal laboratory investigations are related to malabsorption, or to nongut organ involvement, and are nonspecific. Of note is that patients with acquired immune deficiency syndrome (AIDS) with intestinal infection with *Mycobacterium avium intracellulare* (MAI) show infiltration of the lamina propria with PAS-positive macrophages which may mimic Whipple's disease. The Whipple's bacillus and MAI are distinguished by acid-fast staining of the latter.

Notes

MANAGEMENT

Effective antibiotic therapy leads to clinical improvement within a few days and weight gain in 1–2 weeks. The intestinal mucosa may take several months to return to normal. Central nervous system involvement may also be slow to respond and recovery may be incomplete. Relapses are common and therapy needs to be given for at least 12 months. There should subsequently be regular follow-up and repeat small intestinal biopsies.

Of note is that neurologic relapses may occur despite apparently successful eradication of the bacillus from other organs. This is probably because of some inadequate blood–brain barrier penetration of the antibiotics used.

Currently recommended therapy is parenteral penicillin, 1.2 megaunits daily, and streptomycin 1 g daily for 10–14 days. This is followed by *co-trimoxazole* (trimethoprim–sulphamethoxazole) 160/800 mg orally, twice daily for 12 months. Other effective antibiotics are ampicillin, chloramphenicol, doxycycline, erythromycin, and tetracycline. Relapses are treated as for initial therapy.

Other therapy is directed towards the correction of malabsorptive associated deficiencies (see *1.4.9 Overview of Malabsorption*).

1.4.14

Short Bowel Syndrome

Resection of 50% or more of small intestine usually results in significant malabsorption. If only 25% or less

Notes

remains, nutritional support is essential. This support can be either parenteral, enteral, or a combination of both, depending on the severity of malabsorption and the degree of adaptation which slowly develops.

EPIDEMIOLOGY AND PATHOGENESIS

Most commonly, extensive small bowel resection is required when blood supply is compromised. This may occur with superior mesenteric artery thrombosis or embolus, superior mesenteric vein thrombosis, reduced flow in associated arterial or venous branches, small intestinal volvulus, and strangulated internal or external hernias. Other less common causes for extensive resection include Crohn's disease, neoplasia, and trauma.

The severity of the absorptive deficit depends on the extent of resection and the region of resection. Resection of mid small intestine or jejunum is better tolerated than duodenal or ileal resection. Loss of the ileocecal valve will have further detrimental effects because of bacterial contamination of residual small intestine and reduced transit time.

After extensive resection there is a reduction in absorption of virtually all nutrients, including water, electrolytes, carbohydrate, fat, protein, vitamins, and trace elements. This may result in substantial fluid losses, especially for the first few days. Malabsorption may be further exacerbated by transient gastric hypersecretion.

Iron, folate, and calcium are best absorbed in the duodenum and proximal jejunum. Loss of these regions is more likely to predispose to deficiency of these nutrients. Additionally, there is reduced cholecystokinin

Notes

and secretin production with proximal small bowel resection which may result in pancreatic exocrine impairment.

The terminal ileum is the specific site for bile salt and vitamin B_{12} absorption. Resection of less than 100 cm is frequently associated with bile salt malabsorption. Consequent colonic bile salt "overflow" may result in watery diarrhoea (*cholerrheic diarrhoea*), because of reduced absorption and active secretion of fluid and electrolytes. If greater than 100 cm of ileum is resected, absorption is inadequate to maintain the bile salt pool leading to fat malabsorption and steatorrhoea. The degree of vitamin B_{12} malabsorption is also dependent on the length resected.

The remaining small bowel, after resection, undergoes adaptive changes with dilatation, and crypt and villus height increase, leading to increased absorptive area. These changes, however, are slow and may take over a year before maximum effect is reached. Important factors that promote adaptation are pancreaticobiliary secretions, gut hormones, and luminal nutrients. Thus the extent and content of enteral supplementation may influence the degree of adaptation. Potentially important supplements to enteral feeds include pectin, short-chain triglycerides, free fatty acids, and glutamine. These nutrients enhance adaptation in experimental animals; however, experience in humans is limited.

PRESENTATION

Fluid and electrolyte loss, and their manifestations, are the initial features of short bowel syndrome. Subsequently, impaired absorption of other nutrients rapidly

Notes

develops with clinical features of panmalabsorption (see *1.4.9 Overview of Malabsorption*).

An uncommon, but potentially serious, problem, which may be associated with enteral feeding in patients with short bowel syndrome, is recurrent lactic acidosis. Carbohydrate, which is not absorbed in the small intestine, is fermented in the colon to lactate when lactobacilli are present. Treatment is usually with broad-spectrum antibiotics.

INVESTIGATIONS

Initial investigations are directed at maintaining an adequate fluid and electrolyte balance, and include regular biochemistry, daily weighing, and monitoring of fluid loss and replacement. Hypokalemia, hyponatremia, and water depletion are common. Calcium, magnesium, and zinc depletion may also be significant early features. Subsequent laboratory abnormalities are those associated with panmalabsorption (see *1.4.9*) with some variability dependent on the region of resection.

MANAGEMENT

Vigorous parenteral fluid and electrolyte replacement will usually be required for at least a few weeks. Central parenteral nutrition should be initiated early and maintained while diarrhoea remains inadequately controlled. Adult requirements of 2000–3000 kcal per day can be accomplished with amino acid and glucose, and lipid solutions. Iron and vitamin K are not routinely added to parenteral solutions, but can be replaced parenterally (see

Notes

1.4.9). Other trace elements and vitamins can be added to commercial nutritional solutions according to need.

There are a number of drugs that may be used to control diarrhoea (see *Table 23*). When diarrhoea is not troublesome, enteral feeding should be commenced. Parenteral nutrition should be continued, albeit reduced, until the patient can tolerate enteral feeding. It is important to begin enteral feeding early, to stimulate intestinal adaptive hyperplasia.

A formula-defined elemental diet (e.g. Vivonex TEN) may be the most effective way of establishing enteral feeds. Elemental diets contain basic nutrients in monomeric forms which are easier to absorb. Such solutions

Table 23 Drugs used in short bowel syndrome and the reason for their use.

Opioids (see *2.2.1.3*)	To prolong transit and reduce fluid and electrolyte loss
Cholestyramine (4–16 g per day)	To bind bile salts and reduce cholerrheic diarrhoea
Acid suppression H_2 antagonist (ranitidine 150 mg b.i.d.) *or* Proton pump inhibitor (omeprazole 20 mg *mane*)	To reduce gastric hypersecretion and to reduce inactivation of pancreatic enzyme supplements
Pancreatic enzyme replacement (see *2.3.3*)	For pancreatic exocrine impairment
Broad-spectrum antibiotics (see *1.4.15 Bacterial Overgrowth*)	To reduce bacterial contamination of the small bowel or colonic lactobacilli

Notes

are hypertonic and should be diluted to minimize exacerbation of diarrhoea. Formula-defined solutions, however, are unpalatable and may require administration via a thin-bore nasogastric tube. If prolonged tube feeding is needed (> 6 weeks), placement of a feeding tube gastrostomy or jejunostomy should be undertaken. This is usually done percutaneously with endoscopic assistance (percutaneous endoscopic gastrostomy or jejunostomy (PEG or PEJ)).

Patients should be given a trial of solid foods with fat restriction. Small volume, but frequent, meals can be well tolerated. Dietary supplements may be needed, as in other patients with severe malabsorption (see *1.4.9 Overview of Malabsorption*).

Once a patient can tolerate two thirds or more of their caloric intake via elemental feeds, they can usually be converted to polymeric protein-based formulations which contain a substantial amount of fat. Polymeric solutions are better tolerated orally than enteral solutions, and may enable tube feeds to be ceased.

Long-term requirements will be determined by the region of resection, the amount resected, and the degree of adaptation.

1.4.15

Bacterial Overgrowth (Blind Loop Syndrome)

Bacterial overgrowth in the small intestine may occur when there is anatomic abnormality or disordered motility (*Table 24*). This can result in significant malabsorption.

Notes

Table 24 Conditions associated with bacterial overgrowth

- Decreased gastric secretion (especially when combined with anatomic or motility disturbance)
  - Pernicious anaemia
  - Gastric surgery
  - H_2 antagonist or proton pump inhibitor therapy
- Stasis due to anatomic abnormality
  - Afferent loop of Billroth II gastrectomy
  - Other surgically created loops (end-to-side or side-to-side anastomosis)
- Duodenal or jejunal diverticulosis
  - Small intestinal obstruction (stricture, adhesions, inflammation, malignancy)
- Stasis due to motility abnormality
  - Scleroderma
  - Diabetic autonomic neuropathy
  - Intestinal pseudo-obstruction
- Abnormal communication between upper and lower gastrointestinal tract
  - Gastrocolic or enterocolic fistula
  - Resection of the ileocecal valve
- Other
  - Hypogammaglobulinemia (IgA deficiency, congenital and acquired T- and B-cell deficiency, HIV disease)
  - Chronic pancreatitis
  - Irradiation
  - Chronic malnutrition

Terms that have been applied to it include "blind loop syndrome", "stagnant loop syndrome", and "stasis syndrome".

Notes

EPIDEMIOLOGY AND PATHOGENESIS

The normal small bowel flora are Gram-positive organisms at low concentrations, normally maintained by gastric acid and pepsin secretion and by small intestinal motility. When bacterial overgrowth is present the count is high and the flora resembles that of the colon with coliforms and anaerobes.

The effects of bacterial overgrowth are deconjugation and dehydroxylation of conjugated bile leading to fat malabsorption, steatorrhoea, and impaired water and electrolyte transport; hydroxylation of fatty acids, which may be partly responsible for diarrhoea; mild epithelial damage due to the direct toxic effect of deconjugated bile salts; impaired absorption of vitamin B_{12} because of bacterial uptake; and protein and carbohydrate malabsorption. Folate and other vitamin malabsorption, apart from vitamin D, is uncommon because of synthesis by bacteria.

PRESENTATION

The clinical features at presentation are variable and depend on the nature of the underlying cause of the bacterial overgrowth. Blind loop syndrome should be considered in the differential diagnosis of a patient with diarrhoea, steatorrhoea, weight loss, or macrocytic anaemia, especially if they are elderly or have had previous abdominal surgery. If there is a small intestinal stricture, abdominal pain and bloating may be an associated feature.

Notes

INVESTIGATIONS

Small intestinal radiology will demonstrate most anatomic causes of bacterial overgrowth. Standard tests for malabsorption may demonstrate steatorrhoea, impaired xylose excretion, and excessive breath hydrogen production after oral intake of glucose or lactulose (see *1.4.9 Overview of Malabsorption*). Some patients with bacterial overgrowth may have raised fasting levels of breath hydrogen. A Shilling's test for vitamin B_{12} absorption may be abnormal and not corrected by intrinsic factor.

Breath tests utilizing ^{14}C-glycocholic acid or ^{14}C-xylose may be used to diagnose bacterial overgrowth. After ^{14}C-glycocholic acid is administered orally, anaerobic bacterial hydrolysis liberates glycine which is metabolized to $^{14}CO_2$, which is absorbed and detectable in the breath. Normally there is little exhaled $^{14}CO_2$; however, patients with bacterial overgrowth or bile salt malabsorption exhale a substantial amount within 4 hours. The ^{14}C-xylose breath test appears to be more sensitive and specific for bacterial overgrowth. This is partly because it is predominantly absorbed in the proximal rather than distal small intestine.

More complex tests involve duodenal, jejunal, and ileal aspiration with bacterial counts (usually more than 10^5 organisms per ml in blind loop syndrome), aerobic and anaerobic culture, and analysis for unconjugated bile acids or volatile fatty acids.

MANAGEMENT

Malabsorption should be correctable by oral broad-spectrum antibiotics. Tetracycline is the antibiotic of

Notes

choice with improvement usually occurring within a few days. The dose is 250 mg four times a day for 7–10 days repeated every 4–6 weeks, or as symptoms recur. Occasionally, continuous therapy may be needed for months or in the long term.

Other effective antibiotics are the combined use of a cephalosporin (e.g. cephalexin) 250 mg four times a day and metronidazole 200–250 mg three times a day. Alternatively, chloramphenicol (50 mg per kg per day in four divided doses) may be used. The duration of therapy with these other antibiotics is similar to that employed with tetracycline. Rather than repeated courses of the same medication, another approach is use of the different antibiotics in rotation.

Nutritional abnormalities should be corrected (see *1.4.9 Overview of Malabsorption*). If vitamin B_{12} deficiency is the only manifestation of bacterial overgrowth then antibiotics need not be given. Some patients may require enteral or parenteral nutrition either short or long term. Symptomatic therapy may require antidiarrhoeal medication (see *2.2.1 Antidiarrhoeals*).

Specific therapy may be appropriate for some individual disorders such as hypogammaglobulinemia and the diabetic patient with autonomic neuropathy (see *1.4.16 Diabetic Diarrhoea*). Motility stimulants may be tried in intestinal pseudo-obstruction, but are frequently disappointing.

Single or localized anatomic abnormalities may be corrected by surgery. Best results will be achieved if malnutrition can be corrected before an operative procedure. The lesions causing bacterial overgrowth that are amenable to surgery, however, are few.

Notes

1.4.16

Diabetic Diarrhoea

EPIDEMIOLOGY AND PATHOGENESIS

Chronic diarrhoea may be a difficult management problem in 10–20% of insulin-dependent diabetics of long duration.

Several mechanisms may be involved in the pathophysiology. These include visceral autonomic neuropathy with disordered gastrointestinal motility and mucosal electrolyte and fluid transport, bacterial overgrowth, pancreatic exocrine insufficiency, bile salt malabsorption, electrolyte imbalance, and altered gastrointestinal hormone production. Some of the changes associated with the visceral autonomic neuropathy may be secondary to reduced activation of α-adrenergic receptors on enterocytes. Additionally, a point of note is that coeliac disease is more common in type 1 diabetics and requires exclusion.

PRESENTATION

The typical patient with diabetic diarrhoea has longstanding insulin-dependent diabetes that has often been poorly controlled. There are usually associated diabetic complications such as atherosclerosis, retinopathy, glomerulosclerosis, and peripheral neuropathy. Signs of autonomic neuropathy are present, including orthostatic hypotension, neurogenic bladder, anhidrosis or dyshydrosis (e.g. gustatory sweating), and erectile impotence.

The diarrhoea is usually watery, intermittent, and voluminous. It is particularly troublesome at night. Faecal

Notes

incontinence also occurs frequently. When steatorrhoea is present the stool may be bulky.

INVESTIGATIONS

Diabetic diarrhoea is a diagnosis of exclusion. Investigation should rule out remediable causes, especially *infections, chronic pancreatitis, bacterial overgrowth,* and *coeliac disease* (see appropriate sections).

Radiology of the small intestine may show nonspecific dilatation, especially if hypokalemia is present. Radionucleotide studies will usually demonstrate delayed gastric emptying to both liquids and solids ("diabetic gastropathy"). Small bowel transit studies are not helpful in the diagnosis.

Cardiovascular reflex tests may be useful to demonstrate the presence of autonomic nerve dysfunction. These include the absence of change in heart rate and electrocardiograph R–R interval during inspiration and Valsalva maneuvre.

A simple test for autonomic neuropathy is abolition of skin wrinkling of the fingers after water immersion (40°C for 20 min) which occurs when sympathetic function is impaired.

MANAGEMENT

The mainstay of therapy is often opioid antidiarrhoeal agents (see *2.2.1.3 Opioids*). Satisfactory control, however, may not be achieved with such medication.

Case studies has suggested that the α_2 antagonist clonidine may be effective in some patients with diabetic

Notes

diarrhoea. Clonidine is commenced at 100 mg orally 12-hourly and increased to 500 or 600 mg 12-hourly over 3 days. Patients tolerate rather large doses without significant hypotension, possibly because of their autonomic neuropathy. Withdrawal symptoms, however, may be experienced if there is abrupt cessation of clonidine therapy.

An alternative to clonidine is octreotide. Case studies have demonstrated octreotide to be effective in high-volume diabetic diarrhoea, even where clonidine appears not to be effective. Improvement in postural hypotension and a reduction in insulin requirements have also been seen. Octreotide is administered subcutaneously two to four times per day at a total daily dose of 150–300 mg.

1.4.17

Secretory Diarrhoea

Secretory diarrhoea is characterized by high-volume output (more than 1 litre per day) of watery stool that is iso-osmotic to plasma. Most of the causes of secretory diarrhoea (*Table 25*) are discussed elsewhere in this book. The hormone-producing tumours will be the main consideration of this section.

EPIDEMIOLOGY AND PATHOGENESIS

Secretory diarrhoea results from the net secretion of electrolytes and water by the small intestine or colon. This is caused by abnormalities in mucosal ion transport that are partly mediated by intracellular changes in Ca^{2+},

Notes

Table 25 Causes of secretory diarrhoea

Surreptitious laxative or diuretic abuse Stimulant laxatives (see *2.2.4 Laxatives*), docusate sodium, magnesium salts Diarrhoea is a potential dose-related adverse symptom with most diuretics
Bile salt or fatty acid malabsorption
Enterotoxin-associated infectious diarrhoea
Intestinal parasites
Intestinal tuberculosis
HIV-associated enteropathy
Collagen vascular diseases Scleroderma, mixed connective tissue disease, systemic lupus erythematosus
Intestinal lymphoma
Inflammatory bowel disease
Colonic carcinoma or villus adenoma
Microscopic colitis
Hormone-producing tumours Watery diarrhoea, hypokalemia, achlorhydria syndrome (WDHA) Malignant carcinoid syndrome Zollinger–Ellison syndrome Medullary carcinoma of the thyroid
Congenital defects of ion transport

cyclic adenosine monophosphate (AMP) and cyclic guanosine monophosphate (GMP); such as, Na^+-dependent Cl^- secretion by crypt cells, and inhibition of villous brush border Na^+ and Cl^- cotransport. NaCl absorption by the glucose carrier mechanism remains

Notes

intact and is the basis of treatment of watery diarrhoeas with glucose–electrolyte solutions (see *2.2.2 Oral Rehydration Solutions*).

In *WDHA syndrome* (Verner Morrison Syndrome, pancreatic cholera syndrome, VIPoma) the diarrhoea is due to tumour-derived high circulating levels of intestinal secretagogues such as vasoactive intestinal peptide (VIP). The level of another hormone, pancreatic polypeptide, is also often increased in plasma in WDHA syndrome.

The hormone-producing tumour in WDHA syndrome is usually located in the mid or distal pancreas. Most are malignant with metastases at the time of diagnosis. Some VIP-producing primary tumours, such as ganglioneuroblastomas and pheochromocytomas, are found outside the gastrointestinal tract.

In *malignant carcinoid syndrome* the diarrhoea is one component of a multitude of symptoms (see Presentation below). It is due to excessive secretion of serotonin and other peptides or neurotransmitters. Biologically active substances that may be released include histamine, tachykinins (such as substance P), bradykinin, prostaglandins, gastrin, insulin, calcitonin, VIP, adrenocorticotropic hormone (ACTH), and growth hormone- and corticotropin-releasing factors.

Carcinoid tumours may occur anywhere in the gastrointestinal tract from the oesophagus to the rectum, especially in the appendix, small bowel and rectum. The carcinoid syndrome, however, is associated with only a small minority of these tumours, but is noted most frequently with small intestinal carcinoids (approximately 30%), and usually occurs only after extensive metastases to the liver. Other tumours that may produce

Notes

the carcinoid syndrome include bronchial carcinoids, ovarian teratomas, medullary carcinoma of the thyroid, bronchial oat-cell tumours, and common bile duct or pancreatic islet tumours.

The diarrhoea in *Zollinger–Ellison syndrome* is due to excessive amounts of acidic gastric fluid in the small intestine, which interferes with absorption. Small intestinal hyperacidity may inactivate pancreatic lipase resulting in steatorrhoea. The hypersecretion of acid is caused by excessive tumour (gastrinoma) secretion of gastrin. Most gastrinomas arise in the pancreas, especially the pancreatic head. The next most common site is the duodenum. Occurrence in other sites, such as stomach, jejunum, and biliary tree, is rare. At least half are multiple and about two thirds are malignant. Metastatic sites include lymph nodes, liver, spleen, peritoneum, mediastinum, bone, and skin. About one quarter to one third of patients with a gastrinoma have multiple endocrine neoplasia syndrome type I (MEN I), which is characterized by tumours or hyperplasia of the pancreas, parathyroid, and pituitary.

In *medullary carcinoma of the thyroid* the release of calcitonin causes excessive intestinal secretion. Other secretagogues that may be released and contribute to the diarrhoea are prostaglandins, VIP, and, rarely, serotonin (5-hydroxytryptamine, 5-HT). Medullary carcinoma of the thyroid may occur in association with parathyroid hyperplasia and pheochromocytoma (MEN IIa).

PRESENTATION

In most patients the diarrhoea is watery and lacks pus, blood or excessive fat. Stool volume usually ranges

Notes

between 1 and 10 litres per day; excessive secretagogues are more likely to be associated with output at the upper end of the range. Output is not markedly altered by food and usually persists in spite of prolonged fasting (48–72 hours). Exceptions include fatty acid malabsorption and laxative abuse in which the diarrhoea may stop with fasting.

Bicarbonate and potassium are lost in faecal fluid leading to hypokalemia and hyperchloremic metabolic acidosis. The hypokalemia, if severe and persistent, may be associated with extreme weakness and ileus. Volume loss can result in dehydration, hypovolemia, and shock.

There may be specific features on history or examination of the underlying disease, which are evident at presentation and give a clue to the diagnosis. As regards hormone-producing tumours, other features of *WDHA syndrome* are hypochlorhydria, hyperglycemia, hypercalcemia, abnormal glucose tolerance, and flushing; other manifestations of *malignant carcinoid syndrome* may include facial swelling and flushing of upper body, palpitations, metastatic liver enlargement, wheezing, valvular heart disease, and severe weight loss; in *Zollinger–Ellison syndrome* there is usually peptic ulceration, which is resistant to healing, and severe esophagitis; and in *medullary carcinoma of the thyroid* there may be dysphagia due to oesophageal compression and symptoms related to associated tumours (MEN IIa). In many of these tumours, abdominal pain may be a significant feature. This may be due to hypercalcemia, metastatic liver disease, peptic ulceration, increased intestinal motility, intestinal obstruction, and intestinal necrosis.

Notes

INVESTIGATIONS

In secretory diarrhoea the stool osmolality is essentially equal to the concentration of its normal ionic constituents, estimated by $([Na^+]+[K^+]) \times 2$ (multiplied by 2 to account for anions), which is close to the osmolality of plasma. If there is a large osmotic gap (faecal osmolality (measured by freezing point depression) less estimated osmolality), secretory diarrhoea cannot be the only mechanism involved (osmotic gap >50 mOsmol, possible combined secretory and osmotic diarrhoea; >100 mOsmol, probable osmotic diarrhoea). Hypo-osmotic stool can only be due to dilution with urine or water.

Infective causes should be excluded by stool culture and examination for ova, cysts, and parasites. Other tests may be necessary for the diagnosis of parasitic infection (see *1.4.5 Intestinal Parasites*). HIV serology and CD4 counts may be important (see *1.4.8 Diarrhoea in HIV Disease*).

Colonoscopy should be undertaken to exclude colonic pathology. If no macroscopic pathology is evident, serial biopsies should be taken to check for watery diarrhoea-colitis syndrome (see *1.4.23 Watery Diarrhoea–Colitis Syndrome*). Other investigations are a barium meal and small bowel follow-through and/or endoscopy with small bowel biopsy. The order of tests is determined by clinical indications.

Laxative abuse may be intermittent and difficult to detect. Some may be detected by addition of alkali to the stool or urine; a pink colour is indicative of phenolphthalein, and a red colour in urine may indicate aloe or aloin. Anthraquinones, bisacodyl, and phenolphthalein may be

Notes

quantitated in urine. Excess faecal sulphate may indicate magnesium sulphate ingestion. Repeated analysis may be necessary. The above tests may also need to be supplemented by a locker search.

If no disease is evident on the above investigations, tests should be undertaken to determine whether there is tumour-related excessive hormone production. Excessive production of 5-HT (serotonin) and its metabolite 5-hydroxyindoleacetic acid (5-HIAA) is a characteristic abnormality of malignant carcinoid tumours. 5-HIAA may be detected in the urine. 5-HT levels may also be determined in whole blood by reverse-phase high-performance liquid chromatography. Radioimmunoassay may be used to examine for excessive production of gastrin, calcitonin, pancreatic polypeptide and VIP.

In *Zollinger–Ellison syndrome,* gastrin secretion is markedly increased by secretin or calcium infusion, but not in response to a standard meal. Similarly, in *medullary carcinoma of the thyroid,* calcitonin secretion can be enhanced by infusion of pentagastrin or calcium or by ingestion of ethanol. Provocative testing of a hormone-producing tumour should be undertaken in consultation with a specialized centre.

Investigations that may be useful in tumour localization, especially if surgery is contemplated, include ultrasonography, computed tomography, magnetic resonance imaging, arteriography, and percutaneous transhepatic portal venous sampling. Small tumours may also be localized by intraoperative ultrasonography.

Notes

MANAGEMENT

Fluid losses, hypokalemia, and acidosis should be corrected initially. Oral rehydration solutions may be sufficient to balance losses (see *2.2.2 Oral Rehydration Solutions*). If not, then parenteral therapy is necessary. Subsequently investigations can be undertaken to delineate a cause for the secretory diarrhoea.

With hormone-producing tumours, drug therapy may be directed at the tumour and at the associated symptoms. Chemotherapeutic agents that may induce prolonged remission are streptozotocin or chlorozotocin in WDHA syndrome; streptozotocin in malignant carcinoid syndrome, and possibly 5-fluorouracil for hepatic metastases; and streptozotocin and 5-fluorouracil in Zollinger–Ellison syndrome. In a few patients with malignant carcinoid syndrome, interferon a has been documented to reduce tumour size and symptoms.

For symptom relief in Zollinger–Ellison syndrome, a proton pump inhibitor, such as omeprazole or lansoprazole, is the medication of choice. With omeprazole, acid secretion can usually be controlled with less than 80 mg per day, although some patients require more than 200 mg daily.

In medullary carcinoma of the thyroid, prostaglandin inhibition with indomethacin (25 mg two or three times daily) may offset the effect of prostaglandins on the gut. Excess calcitonin may be controlled by bromocriptine (inhibits secretion) and L-dopa (inhibits synthesis).

Symptomatic improvement of diarrhoea may be achieved by the use of opioid antidiarrhoeal drugs (see *2.2.1.3 Opioids*). Octreotide has also been used when other

Notes

means have failed. Control of diarrhoea has been achieved in 60–90% of patients with 50–1000 mg per 24 hours administered subcutaneously in divided doses.

Surgery will be curative in only a minority of patients with a hormone-producing tumour. Local excision, rather than more radical surgery, is usually most appropriate. Laparotomy may be necessary to localize some tumours. In WDHA syndrome, if a tumour cannot be found, a distal two thirds pancreatectomy is recommended. Although many have metastases at the time of diagnosis, surgery is often still indicated because both primary and secondary tumours are usually slow growing, with patients often surviving many years with metastatic disease. Palliative surgical measures include debulking to reduce hormonal secretion and to make conditions more amenable to chemotherapy; in Zollinger–Ellison syndrome, highly selective vagotomy is appropriate at the time of a laparotomy, or total gastrectomy with Roux-en-Y anastomosis if medical therapy has failed; or in malignant carcinoid syndrome, liver transplantation may be indicated because of debilitating symptoms due either to hormonal excess or to hepatic discomfort secondary to metastatic liver disease.

1.4.18

Irritable Bowel Syndrome

Irritable bowel syndrome (IBS) is a common chronic bowel disorder in which abdominal pain is associated with altered bowel habit and abdominal distension in the absence of identifiable disease. IBS is often episodic and

Notes

varies in severity. Unfortunately, in IBS no overall management strategy or drug treatment is globally effective.

EPIDEMIOLOGY AND PATHOGENESIS

Irritable bowel syndrome is present in about 15% of adults, about one quarter of whom will seek medical attention. Half of those with IBS are younger than 35 years, with women presenting two to three times more often than men. Some women experience a worsening of IBS symptomatology during menstruation.

Irritable bowel syndrome is primarily a motor disorder of the gastrointestinal tract, rather than a psychologic disorder. In IBS there is a tendency for hyperreactivity of both the small and large intestine to a variety of stimuli including psychologic stress, drugs, gut peptides, food, and balloon distension. There may also be symptoms associated with smooth muscle dysfunction elsewhere; especially urinary, uterine, or biliary symptoms. Of note, however, is that psychologic factors, especially stressful or threatening life events, influence how people with IBS perceive the symptoms and whether or not they seek medical attention.

PRESENTATION

Symptom criteria for IBS are continuous or recurrent symptoms of:

(a) abdominal pain or discomfort relieved by defaecation and/or associated with a change in stool frequency or consistency; and

Notes

(b) three or more of the following, at least a quarter of the time:
   1 altered stool frequency (more than three bowel movements per day or less than three bowel movements per week)
   2 altered stool form (lumpy/hard or loose/watery)
   3 altered stool passage (straining or urgency, or feeling of incomplete evacuation)
   4 passage of mucus
   5 bloating or feeling of abdominal distension.

Symptoms often occur in discrete episodes which vary in frequency and severity.

Oesophageal and upper gastrointestinal symptoms (e.g. dysphagia, nausea, dyspepsia, and biliary symptoms) often occur in patients with IBS. Extraintestinal symptoms, such as back pain, lethargy, headaches, bladder disturbances, and dyspareunia, are also common.

INVESTIGATIONS

A careful history and physical examination including sigmoidoscopy often enables a confident accurate diagnosis. As part of the initial assessment a dietary history should be taken. Meals high in fat slow gut transit and may be associated with bloating and constipation. Lactose and lactose-containing foods can cause abdominal distension and diarrhoea. Wheat, bran, and their products may cause similar symptoms. High intake of vegetable fiber may also cause discomfort and wind. Sorbitol which is present in many fruits and used as an additive may cause diarrhoea. Fruit juice intake with its

Notes

high fructose and sorbitol content (especially apple or pear juice) may be associated with gas, cramps, and loose bowels. A food diary may help delineate matters further.

IBS cannot be proven directly by investigation. Laboratory and other diagnostic tests are done primarily to rule out other disorders and should be individualized, and care should be taken to avoid excessive investigation. Appropriate initial tests include a complete blood picture, erythrocyte sedimentation rate, stool examination for ova and parasites and fat (if diarrhoea), faecal occult blood examination (if not undertaking other imaging), and rectal biopsy at sigmoidoscopy (if diarrhoea). If there are any symptoms that suggest organic disease such as bleeding, anaemia, fever, weight loss, or recent change in bowel habit, or the patient is aged over 40 years and symptoms are of recent onset, colonoscopy or flexible sigmoidoscopy/barium enema is warranted.

MANAGEMENT

Management is based primarily on the establishment of a positive diagnosis with reassurance of the patient that there is no serious organic disease. There should be explanation that IBS is a genuine clinical entity; that symptoms can wax and wane; that stress may be a major precipitant; and that it will not lead to organic disease. Ongoing review may be important to provide further reassurance and to minimize excessive investigation. If stress appears to be playing a major role then benefit may be obtained by psychologic intervention to assist with stress management and relaxation. Other treatment is dependent on the severity and type of the dominant

Notes

symptoms and includes dietary manipulation and pharmacotherapy.

If any dietary constituents are identified that exacerbate symptoms, they should be avoided. Most patients should have a trial of increased dietary fiber. This should initially be increased gradually and taken with an adequate amount of fluid. If not, there may be an initial exacerbation of IBS-like symptoms. The increased fiber can be in the form of fiber-rich foods or by the use of bulking supplements, especially those that contain *ispaghula* or *psyllium*, which are less likely to cause flatulence. Those benefiting most from fiber supplementation are patients in whom the predominant symptom is constipation; however, those with irregular or alternating bowel habit may also benefit.

There is no pharmacotherapy which is globally effective in IBS. Nevertheless medications may be useful for the control of specific symptoms. For predominant constipation, in addition to dietary changes and exercise, *osmotic laxatives* (lactulose 10–20 ml or more daily) are often effective. For predominant diarrhoea, *loperamide* (up to 8 mg per day in divided doses) may be effective. *Anticholinergic drugs* (dicyclomine 10–40 mg three or four times daily, hyoscine butylbromide 10–20 mg three or four times daily, belladonna herb 45–90 mg three or four times daily), or other *antispasmodic drugs* (mebeverine 135 mg before meals, peppermint oil 0.2 ml before meals) may be useful for intermittent episodes of pain. Anticholinergic or antispasmodic therapy is best taken about half an hour before meals. Anticholinergics often need to be given in doses that cause a dry mouth (xerostomia) before they are clinically effective. A particular concern is

Notes

the side-effects associated with anticholinergics, especially in the elderly, such as urinary retention, blurred vision, and insomnia. In most instances the above drugs need be used only at times of symptom exacerbation. If there is chronic pain, a low dose of an *antidepressant* (e.g. amitriptyline 10 mg *nocte*) can be useful. If significant depression is present, however, full antidepressant therapy is appropriate.

1.4.19

Constipation

Constipation is a symptom that may be defined as infrequent bowel action or difficult or painful defecation. Stool frequency is the easiest parameter to quantify. In normal subjects in Western countries, defecation ranges from three times per day to three times per week. Symptoms such as stool hardness, difficulty in expelling stool, or stool size are difficult to quantify.

EPIDEMIOLOGY AND PATHOGENESIS

The prevalence of constipation varies from 5% to 20% of the population depending on the definition used. In children, boys are more often constipated than girls. This reverses later in life with constipation being more common in females.

Most cases of constipation are due primarily to inadequate dietary fiber and may be termed "simple" constipation. Such people have normal intestinal transit if fiber intake is adequate. Other contributory factors may

Notes

be neglect of the call to stool, unfavorable living or working conditions, and lack of exercise.

Constipation may be secondary to anal, rectal, or colonic disorder such as anorectal fissures, rectal stricture, neoplasia, diverticular disease, inflammatory bowel disease, and motility disorders including irritable bowel syndrome, spastic pelvic floor syndrome (anismus), and descending perineum syndrome.

There are also a number of systemic disorders in which constipation may be a significant problem. These include metabolic disorders such as diabetes, uremia, hypokalemia, and amyloidosis; endocrine disorders including panhypopituitarism, hypothyroidism, hypercalcemia, and pheochromocytoma; scleroderma; and central or peripheral neurologic disorders, for example multiple sclerosis, Parkinson's disease, myotonic dystrophy, cerebrovascular accidents, meningocele, or autonomic neuropathy.

Drugs that may cause constipation include analgesics, antacids (calcium and aluminum compounds), anticholinergics, anticonvulsants, antidepressants, and psychotropic drugs (monoamine oxidase inhibitors), antiparkinsonian drugs, bismuth, diuretics, ganglionic blockers, hypotensives, iron, and opioids.

Chronic stimulant laxative use may lead to worsening constipation because of damage to the myenteric plexus with development of an inert, dilated, aperistaltic colon ("cathartic colon"). The right colon and terminal ileum are usually the most affected region with changes extending more distally in more severe cases. The colonic changes are partially reversible with cessation of the stimulant laxative.

Patients with long-standing severe constipation may have disordered anal function or colonic motility (slow

Notes

transit constipation or colonic inertia). Slow transit constipation and colonic inertia are usually found in women, and begin around the age of puberty. The large bowel may be normal in size and configuration. The constipation can be so severe, however, that it may lead to colectomy. The underlying causes are unknown.

In the elderly, other causes of constipation include immobility, chronic illness, poor nutrition, and reduced fluid intake. Colonic transit studies in elderly constipated patients have shown that the main hold-up is in the rectosigmoid region. This has been termed the *terminal reservoir syndrome* and is an important cause of overflow faecal incontinence.

Chronic constipation, especially in children and the elderly, may lead to faecal impaction in which the rectum becomes distended by a large mass of firm feces which the patient cannot expel. Impaction may be associated with overflow incontinence or ulceration of colonic mucosa (stercoral ulceration).

A less common problem of chronic constipation of any cause is the development of a megacolon. In megacolon the colon enlarges such that the diameter of the rectosigmoid colon is greater than 6.5 cm. It is most commonly found in children or the elderly. In adults megacolon surgery is often necessary. In children there is usually paradoxical contraction of the external anal sphincter during straining which leads to inadequate evacuation. This can often be managed with osmotic laxatives. If there is a history of constipation in the first year of life, Hirschsprung's disease (congenital megacolon) should be considered. In Hirschsprung's disease there is abnormal neuronal development (aganglionosis)

Notes

in the colonic intramural plexuses, beginning at the internal anal sphincter and extending a variable distance proximally. The aganglionic segment is permanently contracted leading to proximal dilatation. Most cases present shortly after birth; however, if the segment involved is very short, symptoms may not develop until after infancy.

PRESENTATION

It is important initially to define what the patient means by their complaint. This will help to determine the most appropriate investigations and management of symptoms.

A key issue at presentation is the duration of symptoms. Constipation since infancy may be due to congenital disease, such as Hirschsprung's disease or meningocele. In later life, recent onset of constipation is often due to significant pathology. Frequently of concern is the possible presence of colonic malignancy. If symptoms have been present for 2 years or more, this is unlikely.

Other factors in the history that need to be considered are associated symptoms, diet, activity, stress, laxative use, drugs that may cause constipation, and the possibility of a systemic disorder.

INVESTIGATIONS

What is outlined below assumes that systemic disorders and drugs have been excluded as causes of the constipation.

Notes

On abdominal examination there may be tenderness and possibly a palpable "mass" over loaded regions of the colon, especially in the sigmoid colon. Distension may be evident if there is obstruction or megacolon present. On anal and rectal examination the cutaneous sensation and anal tone should be assessed. The patient should be asked to strain while the finger is in the rectum. Patients with anismus will squeeze. Sigmoidoscopy should be undertaken to detect rectal lesions and melanosis coli, and will allow the appearance of the stool to be noted. Proctoscopy may be appropriate if anal pathology is suspected.

When abdominal pain and distension are present, plain abdominal radiology may demonstrate faecal loading and/or large bowel obstruction. The level of obstruction and the possible cause may be able to be determined.

Depending on associated symptoms, either colonoscopy or barium enema is appropriate if the constipation is of recent onset. The main purpose of such investigation is to exclude organic disease. If there has been rectal blood loss then colonoscopy should be done.

In Hirschsprung's disease, digital rectal examination in the neonate may result in a gush of faecal material with transient relief of obstruction. In the child or young adult, the rectum will be empty on rectal and sigmoidoscopic examination. At barium enema, the involved segment will be narrow with proximal dilatation. A suction rectal biopsy taken about 25 mm above the internal sphincter may be needed for definitive diagnosis.

In chronic idiopathic constipation the next step is the evaluation of colonic transit. This can be done by

Notes

monitoring the passage of orally administered radio-paque markers by daily plain abdominal radiography. The mean transit time in healthy subjects is about 4 days. Such a test will confirm whether constipation is truly present and may document segmental abnormality. Further investigation may include electromyographic studies, especially of the anal sphincter, anal pressure studies, and dynamic evaluation of defecation using radiology or balloons.

MANAGEMENT

For "simple" constipation review of diet, living, or working conditions, and exercise is appropriate. A high-fiber diet with adequate fluid intake should be instituted gradually. This may be supplemented by *bulk-forming laxatives* (see *2.2.4.1*). In more severe cases a stimulant laxative may be used on a temporary basis.

In simple chronic constipation the long-term use of stimulant laxatives should be avoided, if possible, because of side-effects. Unfortunately, many patients are already established on such medication and are reluctant to stop them. In this situation an attempt should be made to minimize their use by prescribing bulk-forming or hyperosmotic laxatives.

In children, if a high-fiber diet and bulk-forming laxatives are not sufficient then a *lubricant* (see *2.2.4.2*) is preferred. An alternative is a hyperosmotic laxative such as lactulose. Stimulant laxatives are preferably avoided in children.

In the immobile patient, increasing bulk is relatively contraindicated in the management of chronic constipa-

Notes

tion. This is because constipation may actually worsen in what may be an already distended colon. The best initial choice of medication is probably a *hyperosmotic laxative* (see *2.2.4.6*). This may need to be supplemented by an enema or suppository twice weekly. Alternatively, the addition of an anthraquinone *stimulant laxative* (see *2.2.4.7*) may be necessary. Other laxatives such as paraffin oil (mineral oil) and phenolphthalein should be avoided because of their potential side-effects.

Severe acute constipation or faecal impaction may initially be managed by enema/washout therapy, using plain water or saline, or phosphate enemas (see *2.2.4.4 Saline Laxatives*). The faecal mass may be softened with 150 ml of olive oil as a retention enema two to four times over 2 days, before washout. An alternative softener is rectally administered docusate (see *2.2.4.3 Stool Softeners*). Soap enemas are harmful and should not be used. Another option is an orally administered *isotonic electrolyte solution* (see *2.2.4.5*). It may take about 1 week to clean the colon and rectum completely. If obstruction is present, manual removal is necessary under general anaesthesia or after narcotic analgesia, such as pethidine 100 mg. Thereafter the above measures should be instituted until the colon is clear. Subsequently treatment should be as for chronic constipation.

It is useful, especially in children, to establish a pattern of regular toileting, most suitably after breakfast to take advantage of the gastrocolic reflex. Behavioral therapy can be used to help establish this. Provision of a footstool and adoption of a forward leaning position on a standard toilet may assist with defaecation in both young and old. In the older patient not responding adequately to simple

Notes

measures, education and functional retraining including biofeedback techniques (e.g. pelvic floor incoordination), or psychological therapy (e.g. irritable bowel syndrome), may be useful. This may require referral to a multidisciplinary team with an interest in this area for assessment and management.

Surgery is the main treatment for Hirschsprung's disease. Other situations in which it may be of use are when outlet obstruction has been demonstrated, in which case anorectal myectomy may be of benefit, and in patients with severe constipation due to colonic inertia where colectomy with ileorectal anastomosis may be appropriate.

1.4.20

Diverticular Disease of the Colon

In diverticular disease of the colon, the basic abnormality is an acquired herniation of the mucosa and submucosa through the muscular wall (diverticulosis). This occurs most frequently in the sigmoid region, but may be found anywhere in the colon. In some there may be associated symptoms and signs of illness (diverticulitis).

EPIDEMIOLOGY AND PATHOGENESIS

Diverticular disease is present in about 5–10% of people in Western countries but is rare in developing countries. About one third to one half of individuals over the age of 60 years have diverticular disease, but it is uncommon before the age of 40 years; females are affected more

Notes

frequently than males. Only about 5% of those with diverticula will develop diverticulitis.

The anatomy of the colon predisposes to the development of diverticula. The longitudinal muscle is grouped into teniae coli and the circular muscle into fascicles, leaving areas of relative weakness. This weakness may be contributed to by age-related molecular changes in collagen. Diverticula develop in these areas of weakness, particularly where nutrient blood vessels pass through to the submucosa. The sigmoid region is the most common area involved (95% of cases).

Diet probably plays a major role in the development of diverticula. There is an inverse relationship between the intake of cereal fiber and the occurrence of diverticular disease ("fiber hypothesis"). The addition of fiber to the diet not only increases the wet weight and diameter of the stool, but also reduces intraluminal pressure and spontaneous motor activity. Colonic hypermotility and increased intraluminal pressure have been noted in some patients with diverticular disease, principally in the sigmoid region, and may be a major factor in diverticula development. Most of these patients have shortening and thickening of the teniae and thickening of circular muscle.

Diverticulitis is the most common complication of diverticulosis. The early pathologic feature is focal inflammation in the wall of a diverticulum at its apex, in response to inspissated faecal material. This inflammation extends to the peridiverticular region with resultant necrosis, microperforation or macroperforation, and faecal contamination of the surrounding tissues. The most common site is the sigmoid region and usually only

Notes

one diverticulum is involved. Usually the inflammation is contained locally. If not, secondary complications such as intra-abdominal abscess, fistula, bowel obstruction, and generalized peritonitis may occur.

PRESENTATION

Only a small subset of people with diverticular disease have symptoms. In uncomplicated (simple) diverticular disease, the most common symptom is intermittent griping pain in the left iliac fossa and suprapubic regions which may persist for a few hours to several days. It may also be worse after eating, and eased by defaecation or the passage of flatus. There may be associated constipation, diarrhoea, or flatulence. The pain may be due to colonic muscular contraction and the associated increased intraluminal pressure. On examination, there may be tenderness over the sigmoid colon on palpation, but no signs of peritonism and no fever. Uncomplicated diverticular disease may be difficult to distinguish from irritable bowel syndrome.

In diverticulitis, not only is there pain and bowel irregularity, but there is frequently fever. Abdominal tenderness may be more marked and peritonism evident. A fixed mass may also be palpable on either abdominal or rectal examination. Bowel sounds may be reduced. Leucocytosis is also a frequent feature. The differential diagnosis includes carcinoma of the colon, Crohn's disease, ulcerative colitis and ischaemic colitis.

Rectal bleeding may occur in about 15% of patients with diverticulosis. The severity ranges from slight to life threatening (5%). Such patients commonly have few

Notes

symptoms before the episode. In many cases the site of bleeding is a single diverticulum in the right colon.

INVESTIGATIONS

When simple diverticular disease is suspected, then sigmoidoscopy and barium enema are appropriate investigations. Radiology is more sensitive than colonoscopy in documenting diverticula.

In diverticulitis, early flexible sigmoidoscopy is important in most cases for the exclusion of other diagnoses and for evaluation of the rectum and lower sigmoid should surgical resection be necessary. A characteristic feature is spasm of the sigmoid colon associated with pain and inability to pass the instrument beyond the rectosigmoid flexure. Radiology is also an important part of the initial evaluation. Plain abdominal radiology may reveal an ileus or obstruction, or free air in the peritoneal cavity associated with perforation. A carefully performed barium enema may be of diagnostic value. Computed tomography can also prove useful in the diagnosis of diverticulitis and its complications.

MANAGEMENT

Diets high in vegetable and cereal fiber relieve pain and associated symptoms. Good results have been achieved with *unprocessed wheat bran* taken in the maximum amount tolerated. This should be built up gradually because of bloating and abdominal discomfort which may be associated with high bran intake. An alternative to bran are *hydrophilic laxatives* (see *2.2.4.1 Bulk-Forming*

Notes

Laxatives). *Antispasmodics* (see 2.2.3), such as mebeverine and trimebutine, may give symptomatic relief. Opiate analgesics such as morphine are contraindicated because they increase intraluminal pressure. Pethidine (meperidine), however, does not appear to have this risk. There is no rationale for the use of antibiotics in the management of uncomplicated diverticular disease.

The initial therapy of diverticulitis is usually medical. If the disease is severe enough to require hospital admission, then appropriate initial treatment measures include bedrest, nil orally and nasogastric suction if bowel obstruction is present, intravenous fluids, analgesia, and antibiotics. In a severe case, a multiple antibiotic drug regimen provides the best cover, albeit with a greater risk of toxicity. An appropriate regimen would be ampicillin 2 g intravenously 6 hourly, gentamicin 4–5 $mg\,kg^{-1}day^{-1}$, either as two divided doses 12 hourly or as a single daily dose, and metronidazole 500 mg intravenously 12 hourly. If gentamicin is contraindicated then either cefotaxime (1 g intravenously 8 hourly) or ceftriaxone (1 g intravenously 24 hourly) could be substituted. For the patient with penicillin hypersensitivity, ampicillin may be omitted, but the remaining combination will not provide full cover. In the less severe case a single broad-spectrum antibiotic may suffice. Possible single regimens are *cefoxitin* 2 g intravenously 8 hourly, cefotetan 2 g intravenously 12 hourly, or ticarcillin/potassium clavulanate 3/0.1 g intravenously 4–6 hourly. Symptoms and signs will usually abate within 3–10 days.

Urgent surgical intervention may be required if there is generalized peritonitis, persistent obstruction unresponsive to medical therapy, or the development or

Notes

persistence of a pericolic abscess despite antimicrobial therapy. Emergency surgery may also be required for persistent colonic bleeding. Elective colonic resection should be considered after the episode if there is a residual fistula or a colonic narrowing in which cancer cannot be excluded. Some patients with recurrent episodes of acute diverticulitis may also benefit from colonic resection.

1.4.21

Colorectal Carcinoma

Sporadic adenocarcinoma of the colourectum is one of the leading causes of death from cancer, especially in developed countries. Worldwide it is the third most common cancer in males and the fourth most common cancer in females.

EPIDEMIOLOGY AND PATHOGENESIS

There is a variable geographic incidence of sporadic colorectal carcinoma, especially distal colonic carcinoma. Incidence rates are highest in Westernized countries. In countries of low incidence of colonic cancer, right-sided lesions predominate; in countries of high incidence, left-sided lesions predominate. Rectal carcinoma tends to follow a similar geographic pattern to left-sided colonic cancer.

Western-style diets which are high in fats, heavily browned fried red meat, and refined carbohydrates, and low in dietary fiber have been associated with colorectal

Notes

cancer. These and other less defined factors predispose to mutational change that alters cellular proliferation, differentiation, and cell death within colonic epithelium. These changes result in increased epithelial growth, leading to adenoma development, and eventually to carcinoma.

Other risk factors include age over 40 years: personal history of colorectal adenoma or carcinoma; family history of a first-degree relative with colorectal cancer, a polyposis syndrome, or nonpolyposis inherited colonic cancer; and inflammatory bowel disease.

A modified Dukes' staging system for colorectal cancer is useful for estimating survival and planning adjuvant therapy. In this classification tumours are designated: A, if limited to the mucosa; B1, if extending into, but not through, the muscularis propria; B2, if penetrating the bowel wall, but no lymph node involvement; C, if there is also regional lymph node involvement with tumour; and 'D', if distant metastases are present. Stage C tumours may be further divided into those in which the primary tumour is limited to the bowel wall (C1) or penetrates the bowel wall (C2). Survival rates (5-year) for Dukes' A tumours range from 70 to 100%. Survival rates for other stages are B1 65%, B2 43%, C1 53% and C2 15%.

PRESENTATION

Symptoms depend to some extent on the location of the primary tumour. The common clinical modes of presentation in order of frequency for left-sided cancer are rectal blood loss (haematochezia), diarrhoea, mucus, pain, and constipation; for right-sided cancers they are pain,

Notes

constipation, diarrhoea, and haematochezia. Because bleeding from right-sided cancers is less apparent, these lesions tend to be larger and more often have associated anaemia.

INVESTIGATIONS

When colorectal cancer is suspected, prompt diagnostic investigation should be undertaken preferably by colonoscopy, or alternatively by flexible sigmoidoscopy and double-contrast barium enema. The latter tests are more sensitive than colonoscopy in determining a cause for rectal blood loss, because of increased detection of diverticula; however, colonoscopy is more sensitive in detecting adenoma and cancer, and allows procedural intervention. If a carcinoma is found radiologically, full colonoscopic examination should be attempted in order to detect synchronous lesions before surgery. If this is not feasible then colonoscopic examination should be undertaken within about 3 months of surgery.

MANAGEMENT

Surgical resection is the appropriate treatment for most patients with colorectal cancer; including those with distant metastases, to prevent obstruction or bleeding. Segmental colonic resection is undertaken with a wide resection margin. The extent is determined by blood supply and lymphatic drainage.

The liver is the most common site of distant metastases in colorectal cancer. These may be synchronous in 10–25% of patients. If there is disease recurrence the liver is involved in 40–70% of patients. If there are fewer than

Notes

four hepatic lesions present, strong consideration should be given to surgical resection. Other methods that may limit the growth of discrete lesions include alcohol injection, cryotherapy, hepatic artery infusion chemotherapy, interstitial laser therapy, and interstitial radiotherapy.

The value of adjuvant therapy is continuing to be evaluated. The aim is to minimize the incidence of tumour recurrence after apparently curative surgery and to improve patient survival. It is of minimal value in the treatment of metastatic disease. Adjuvant radiotherapy, either before or after operation, for rectal carcinoma is under active investigation. Published studies suggest that it may reduce local recurrence but does not appear to alter survival. Current evidence also suggests that adjuvant chemotherapy with 5-fluorouracil (5-FU) and *levamisole* for Dukes' C colonic cancer may be effective in reducing local recurrence and improving disease-free survival. The overall value of adjuvant therapy, however, remains uncertain and it is appropriate that, if it is to be used, it should be within a clinical trial setting.

1.4.22

Inflammatory Bowel Disease (Ulcerative Colitis and Crohn's Disease/Regional Enteritis)

Ulcerative colitis and Crohn's disease are the two major forms of inflammatory bowel disease. Most commonly they have a chronic intermittent course, with periods of remission from months to years.

Notes

Ulcerative colitis is characterized by nonspecific colonic mucosal inflammation which invariably affects the rectum and extends in continuity to involve a variable extent of the proximal colon such that the area involved may be called proctitis, proctosigmoiditis, or distal colitis, left-sided disease, subtotal colitis or total colitis.

Crohn's disease is also a nonspecific inflammatory process, but often involves the full thickness of the bowel wall. It may also affect any part of the gastrointestinal tract. Most commonly, however, it involves the ileocecal region, small bowel, or colon. Disease is usually discontinuous (segmental). When the rectum is involved it may be difficult to distinguish from ulcerative colitis.

EPIDEMIOLOGY AND PATHOGENESIS

The initiating processes in inflammatory bowel disease remain unknown. There are, however, probably genetic predisposing factors, exogenous and endogenous triggers, and modifying factors involved. These lead to a spontaneous relapsing and remitting inflammatory process in which tissue injury is mediated by the immune system; predominantly by nonautoimmune mechanisms including T cell and neutrophil activation.

Most information regarding the occurrence of inflammatory bowel disease is from developed countries. Areas of high incidence or prevalence include Scandinavian countries, the UK, North America, Australia, and New Zealand. It seems less common in southern Europe. The incidence of both ulcerative proctitis and more extensive ulcerative colitis has increased from the 1930s; since

Notes

about 1970, however, the incidence of extensive ulcerative colitis appears to have been decreasing. The incidence of Crohn's disease also increased up to the early 1970s, but appears to have since either stabilized or decreased.

Initial presentation with inflammatory bowel disease appears to be bimodal with peaks in those aged 20–40 and over the age of 60. Sex incidences are very similar below the age of 55 years, but the condition is about 1.5 times more frequent in males over 55. Both Crohn's disease and ulcerative colitis occur more commonly in families than would be expected by chance (positive family history 10–20%). However, the degree to which this is genetic or environmental is uncertain. Patients with ulcerative colitis are likely to be nonsmokers, whereas those with Crohn's disease tend to be smokers and to have an increased sugar intake. A slightly increased risk of Crohn's disease has also been reported with oral contraceptive use.

1.4.22.1

ULCERATIVE COLITIS

PRESENTATION

The clinical presentation of ulcerative colitis is dependent on the extent and severity of the disease. In mild disease there may be either a slight increase in stool frequency (fewer than four daily) or a small amount of blood and mucus evident in the stool, or both. There may also be urgency and mild lower abdominal discomfort that is

Notes

relieved by defecation, but no features of systemic illness. In severe disease there is the passage of six or more bloody stools per day and evidence of systemic illness such as fever, tachycardia, anaemia, and an ESR (erythrocyte sedimentation rate) greater than 30 mm in the first hour. Urgency and pain are more pronounced. Also with severe disease there is usually weight loss, malaise, and lethargy. Moderate disease is intermediate between mild and severe.

INVESTIGATIONS

Checking the diagnosis is a vital initial step in the management of an acute episode of ulcerative colitis. Initial investigations should include faecal microscopy and culture, and analysis for *Clostridium difficile* toxin (see *1.4.7 Antibiotic-Associated Colitis and Pseudomembranous Colitis*). In an endemic area, fresh stool should be examined for amoebae. A plain abdominal radiograph, to exclude colonic dilatation, should be done unless the attack is mild. This may also help assess the extent of the disease with affected bowel being empty of faecal material. Plain abdominal radiology should be repeated daily while mild dilatation remains. Examination may need to be more frequent if there is moderate dilatation. Marked dilatation is an indication for emergency surgery. Radiology should also be repeated if treatment response is slow or there is a deterioration of symptoms.

Laboratory parameters that should be examined include a full blood examination which may reveal anaemia, neutrophilia, and thrombocytosis in moderate to severe disease; urea and electrolytes, and liver

Notes

function tests (a reduced level of albumin may be evident in severe disease); iron stores, which may be low because of blood loss; and red cell folate, the absorption of which may be impaired if on sulphasalazine.

Rigid proctosigmoidoscopy with biopsy is also important in the initial assessment of an acute episode, and in monitoring response to therapy. A barium enema or flexible sigmoidoscopic examination, however, is usually not undertaken in severe active disease because of the risk of perforation or precipitating toxic megacolon.

There are a range of sigmoidoscopic features that match the severity of the disease. The earliest appearances are loss of the normal vascular pattern and mucosal hyperemia and edema. With more severe inflammation, the mucosa becomes granular and eventually friable so that contact results in petechial haemorrhages. In severe colitis, the mucosa bleeds spontaneously and may be frankly ulcerated, and the lumen contains large amounts of reddish-brown liquid (diarrhoea, pus, and blood). The inflammation in ulcerative colitis tends to be homogeneous and to extend proximally from the rectum. In some patients with severe disease, however, injury may be more severe above the rectum. In remission, the mucosa may appear normal. However, with repeated attacks it becomes pale and atrophic.

In the patient who has had ulcerative colitis for 8–10 years, irrespective of severity, a full colonoscopy should be undertaken, with random biopsies taken at intervals around the colon. This is primarily to document the extent of disease. Current recommendations are that patients with disease beyond the sigmoid colon should

---

Notes

participate in a surveillance program with colonoscopy and multiple biopsies every 1–2 years. This is to attempt to detect dysplastic tissue before it develops into carcinoma, the definitive intervention being colectomy.

MANAGEMENT

Therapy in ulcerative colitis is determined mainly by the severity and extent of the disease.

Proctitis and distal colitis

Patients with proctitis or distal colitis may initially be treated with *topical corticosteroids* (*budesonide, hydrocortisone,* or *methylprednisolone*), as either suppository, foam, or enema. Suppositories are suitable for proctitis, foams for limited left-sided disease, and enemas for more extensive disease up to about 60 cm from the anus (to the splenic flexure). Therapy is applied once (or twice) daily for 2 weeks, and then reduced to alternate days (or once daily) for a further fortnight. *Sulphasalazine* or *mesalazine,* suppositories or enemas, are alternative therapies (see *2.2.5 Sulphasalazine* and *2.2.6 Aminosalicylates*), which may also be effective if topical corticosteroids have failed.

Many patients prefer oral to rectal therapy. Oral *sulphasalazine*, or another *aminosalicylate*, is an alternative to rectal therapy in mild disease (see 2.2.5 and 2.2.6). In the patient who is slow to respond or who has more than mild disease, it is appropriate to combine oral and rectal therapy, for example an oral salicylate with rectal corticosteroid. If response remains inadequate (approxi-

Notes

mately 20% of cases), systemic steroids or other immunosuppressive therapy may be necessary (see *Moderate disease* or *Severe disease* below). Rarely, surgery is required.

Some patients with distal disease have abdominal discomfort related to faecal loading proximal to the diseased segment. This usually responds to the use of a bulk-forming laxative (see *1.4.19 Constipation*).

After an initial episode that has responded quickly to therapy, long-term maintenance treatment is not usually indicated. However, if the episode has initially been refractory to treatment, indefinite maintenance therapy is probably appropriate. Long-term maintenance treatment should also be considered if relapses occur frequently or are difficult to treat. The most suitable long-term maintenance therapies are oral or topical aminosalicylates (see *2.2.5* and *2.2.6*). Aminosalicylate enemas or suppositories may be able to maintain remission with use once every few days. Rectal steroids may be similarly used; however, long-term oral steroids are preferably avoided because of potential side-effects.

Disease proximal to the sigmoid colon

Mild disease

For mild disease, initial therapy can be with an oral *sulphasalazine* or other *aminosalicylate*. Steroid or mesalazine enemas may be used as adjunctive therapy. Clinical remission is usually achieved in 3–4 weeks in about 75% of patients. Thereafter, indefinite oral aminosalicylate maintenance therapy is appropriate.

Notes

Moderate disease

Patients with moderate disease, or nonresponsive mild disease, usually respond within a few weeks to oral *corticosteroids* (*prednisone, prednisolone*) at 30–60 mg day^{-1} (1 mg kg^{-1} day^{-1} in children). Oral sulphasalazine or another aminosalicylate may be started at the time of initiating steroids. When satisfactory symptom control is achieved, the corticosteroid can be reduced, initially by 10 mg per week until on 20–25 mg daily, then by 5 mg per week. If there is a relapse, the dose is increased and subsequent tapering is slower.

Some patients become dependent on long-term oral corticosteroids to maintain disease remission. The options then are continued steroid therapy, if only low doses are required; alternative or additional immunosuppressive therapy, such as azathioprine (or 6-mercaptopurine) or methotrexate; or colectomy.

Azathioprine and *6-mercaptopurine* are similar drugs which can be used almost interchangeably. Azathioprine is converted by the body to 6-mercaptopurine. Azathioprine is often started at a dose of 100 mg per day in the average sized adult. It may take 12 weeks or more before it is fully clinically effective. The starting dose corresponds to about 1.5 mg kg^{-1} day^{-1}, which may be increased to 2.5 mg kg^{-1} day^{-1} if response is inadequate. About one in ten patients are not able to tolerate azathioprine or 6-mercaptopurine because of adverse side-effects such as severe nausea, dose-dependent bone marrow suppression (especially leucopenia), fever, pancreatitis (about 3%), and rarely hepatitis. Blood cell counts should be monitored weekly for the first 4–6 weeks, and less frequently thereafter.

Notes

In chronic active ulcerative colitis, azathioprine can help induce remission and enable reduction of the corticosteroid dose in at least two thirds of patients. Azathioprine, however, does not increase the clinical effectiveness of corticosteroids in acute ulcerative colitis. When remission is established, the corticosteroid dose can be tapered and possibly ceased. If effective, azathioprine is usually continued for at least 1 year. About one third of patients will have further relapses on azathioprine which are usually controllable with corticosteroid therapy, as per an acute attack. If the patient has remained in remission, the azathioprine could be stopped. About 60% of patients, however, will have a significant relapse and may require long-term therapy.

Uncontrolled studies have suggested that methotrexate (25 mg intramuscularly, weekly) may also be useful adjunctive therapy in inducing remission. It is effective in about 75% of patients refractory to other therapy. Although it takes some weeks to be clinically effective, its onset of action is more rapid than that of azathioprine.

Severe disease

For severe disease, or nonresponsive moderate disease, admission to hospital and administration of intravenous *corticosteroids* is indicated. Intravenous hydrocortisone 100 mg every 6–8 hours (10 $mg\,kg^{-1}\,day^{-1}$ in children), prednisolone 60–80 mg per day, or methylprednisolone 48–60 mg daily are the main corticosteroids used. Clinical trials have shown that corticotrophin (ACTH), either intramuscular or intravenous, may be as effective as intravenous corticosteroids. ACTH tends not to be

Notes

used, however, because of the unpredictable adrenal response, especially after previous steroid therapy.

In the patient with severe disease, other therapy may include intravenous fluid and electrolytes, blood transfusion, and possibly intravenous nutrition and antibiotics. Intravenous nutrition is usually not necessary, unless oral intake is inadequate because of nausea or vomiting, as there is no evidence that bowel rest is beneficial. Thus patients can be fed unless an emergency colectomy is a possibility. If malnutrition is present, enteral supplementation may be necessary. There is no evidence that antibiotics are of benefit in severe disease unless the patient has a possible infective complication (toxic megacolon with systemic toxicity or peritoneal signs) or is undergoing emergency surgery.

Most patients will respond to intravenous corticosteroids within 5 days. They can then be switched to oral corticosteroids, as for moderate disease. If disease still remains severe, but clinically stable, then a further 5 days of intensive therapy is warranted. If there is deterioration at any stage, or no improvement after 10 days, then surgery is indicated. In the stable, but not improving, patient, in whom surgery is threatening, intravenous cyclosporin may be an additional therapeutic option. Cyclosporin, 4 $mg\,kg^{-1}\,day^{-1}$ as a continuous infusion, may avert colectomy in about 80% of patients not controlled by steroids alone. Use of such medication is not without problems and requires close monitoring.

If there is a satisfactory response to intravenous cyclosporin and corticosteroids the patient can be converted to oral therapy. Oral cyclosporin is given

Notes

twice daily (total daily dose approximately 5 mg kg^{-1}) with adjustment to maintain whole blood trough levels between 150 and 250 μg l^{-1}. Because cyclosporin may be associated with significant adverse side-effects or drug interactions and requires regular monitoring, it should be used in consultation with experienced personnel. Cyclosporin is frequently insufficient in itself to maintain remission; therefore oral corticosteroids are usually not tapered below 10 mg per day. Cyclosporin can be continued for 3–4 months or longer. To make long-term management less complicated, it is preferable to make a gradual switch to azathioprine or methotrexate when the steroid dose is low (at about 2 months) with the view to ceasing cyclosporin when these other agents are theoretically working (after 8–12 weeks for azathioprine, 4 weeks for methotrexate).

1.4.22.2

CROHN'S DISEASE

PRESENTATION

The clinical presentation of Crohn's disease is more variable than that of ulcerative colitis. This variability is related to the area of bowel that is affected. In approximate terms about one third of patients have small bowel disease, one third have small bowel and colonic disease, and one third have only colonic disease. Most of those with small bowel disease have terminal ileal involvement. Colonic disease is usually segmental,

Notes

but occasionally may be pancolonic; it may also be contiguous with the rectum and resemble ulcerative colitis.

A triad of symptoms that is often present is diarrhoea, abdominal pain, and weight loss. The diarrhoea is multifactorial. Stools may be watery because of seepage of fluid from inflamed tissue, because of the colonic effects of bile salt overflow with ileal disease, or occasionally because of enteric fistulae. Steatorrhoea may be present with extensive ileal disease. There may also be malabsorptive diarrhoea with bacterial overgrowth occurring in dilated loops proximal to segmental stricturing of the small bowel. The abdominal pain may be directly related to an inflammatory mass, especially in the right iliac fossa; or could be obstructive in nature with postprandial abdominal discomfort and distension.

Extraintestinal manifestations, such as arthropathy, iritis, erythema nodosum, and pyoderma gangrenosum, may be associated with either Crohn's disease or ulcerative colitis. Features that are usually characteristic of Crohn's disease include ulceration, sepsis, and fistulae of the perianal region.

INVESTIGATIONS

As with ulcerative colitis, faecal specimens should be examined to exclude infective conditions. *Yersinia enterocolitica* (see *1.4.2.2.4*) infection may be difficult to distinguish from early Crohn's disease because of similar symptoms and inflammation of the distal ileum. A rising titre of agglutinating antibodies or demonstration of *Yersinia* in the stool will enable differentiation. Another

Notes

infection which may mimic Crohn's disease is *Mycobacterium tuberculosis*, which can result in segmental small bowel and colonic disease. Gastrointestinal tuberculosis, however, is rare in developed countries.

Radiology or endoscopy with biopsy is often critical for establishing the diagnosis. The colon and terminal ileum can usually be visualized endoscopically. Radiology is necessary for adequate examination of the small bowel. The endoscopic findings described for ulcerative colitis can also occur in Crohn's disease; however, the process is usually discontinuous. Other findings may include aphthous ulcers, deep pleomorphic or serpiginous ulcers, cobblestone mucosa, strictures, and fistulae. Fistulae, if suspected, are better identified radiologically than endoscopically.

Other investigations which may be useful include ultrasonography, computed tomography, and magnetic resonance imaging, especially for detection of abdominal extraluminal problems such as a suspected abdominal abscess. Additionally, an indium- or technetium-labelled neutrophil scan may be a simple effective way of identifying recurrent bowel disease if there is diagnostic uncertainty.

The occasional patient with Crohn's disease only has disease extending from the rectum which can be difficult to distinguish from ulcerative colitis. There may be no extracolonic features or small bowel disease which aid the diagnosis. Biopsies may also be equivocal. Such patients are regarded initially as having "indeterminate colitis".

As with ulcerative colitis, important laboratory parameters that should be examined in acute Crohn's disease

Notes

include a full blood examination, estimation of urea and electrolytes, and liver function tests. The ESR or C-reactive protein level may be a useful guide of disease activity, especially in delineating recurrence or response to therapy. Additionally, serum vitamin B_{12} levels should be determined if ileal disease is suspected.

MANAGEMENT

The management of Crohn's disease depends on the site and extent of disease, the severity of disease, and the complications of the disease. When the large bowel is involved, therapy is often similar to that for ulcerative colitis. Corticosteroids, either rectally, orally, or intravenously, are the mainstay of treatment of moderate to severe active gastrointestinal disease. If response is inadequate, other immunosuppressive therapy, such as azathioprine (or 6-mercaptopurine), cyclosporin, or methotrexate, may be required.

Oral disease

The most common oral lesions are aphthoid ulcers, which usually respond well to a steroid-based mouthwash or paste. If the intention is to treat with systemic corticosteroids because of disease elsewhere, simple pastes such as Orabase are a suitable initial option. In the resistant patient, azathioprine may be required.

Ooesophageal, gastric, and duodenal disease

Proximal gastrointestinal disease often mimics peptic ulcer disease. Symptoms associated with oesophageal

Notes

ulceration are often relieved rapidly by a short course of oral corticosteroids. Many patients with gastroduodenal disease respond satisfactorily to strong acid suppression with high-dose *H_2 antagonists* or a *proton pump inhibitor* (*omeprazole, lansoprazole,* or *pantoprazole*), which may need to be maintained long term. The more difficult patient requires corticosteroids and may need azathioprine.

Ileitis, ileocolitis, and colitis

Sulphasalazine and the other *aminosalicylates* may be effective in the treatment of mild to moderate acute colonic disease and as maintenance therapy. Aminosalicylate preparations that release mesalazine in the small intestine, such as *Asacol* and *Pentasa* (see *2.2.5 Sulphasalazine* and *2.2.6 Aminosalicylates*), are similarly effective in ileal disease. These medications may also reduce the likelihood of postoperative recurrence after ileocolonic resection.

Oral corticosteroids are often the main initial therapy because they are more effective than aminosalicylates in acute disease, and because recurrences that do occur are usually not mild. Although steroids are used in a similar initial dose as in ulcerative colitis (prednisone or prednisolone dosage of 30–60 mg per day (1 mg kg^{-1} day^{-1} in children)), tapering is more gradual with therapy being maintained for 2–3 months or longer.

In severe cases, initial therapy is with intravenous corticosteroids, as in ulcerative colitis. Steroids can be used safely in a patient with an abdominal mass, with frequent good clinical response. Limited experience with

Notes

intravenous cyclosporin has suggested efficacy as adjunctive therapy to steroids in severe disease, especially colonic or fistulous disease (see above *Ulcerative Colitis – Management*). However, in maintaining remission, low-dose oral cyclosporin therapy appears not to be effective.

In ileocecal Crohn's disease a potential short- and long-term option may be Eudragit-coated budesonide. This preparation gives ileal and right-sided colonic release of budesonide, a corticosteroid with high first-pass hepatic clearance. Because of low systemic levels, budesonide is associated with fewer steroid-related side-effects. Recent clinical studies have shown it to have short-term efficacy which approaches that of prednisolone and the ability in the long term to delay relapse compared with placebo. The appropriate dose, however, needs to be defined further.

Often disease recurs after tapering to a low steroid dose or shortly after steroid cessation. In such patients, adjunctive therapy such as aminosalicylates or immunosuppressives (azathioprine, methotrexate) may be necessary with possibly long-term low-dose corticosteroid. In some patients, immunosuppressive therapy, without corticosteroids, is sufficient for maintenance therapy. In others, long-term intermediate doses (prednisolone 10–20 mg per day), although undesirable, are needed to maintain disease control.

Azathioprine (or *6-mercaptopurine*) has similar clinical effectiveness to its action in ulcerative colitis as regards onset, remission induction, and maintenance. It is used in similar doses (see above *Ulcerative Colitis – Management*). Methotrexate (25 mg intramuscularly, weekly) may also be effective therapy in maintaining remission and

Notes

reducing corticosteroid requirements. Lower doses of methotrexate (approximately 15 mg orally) for maintenance therapy of Crohn's disease and ulcerative colitis are currently under investigation.

Perianal or fistulous disease

Metronidazole is the most commonly used antibiotic in Crohn's disease. Its usage, however, has been primarily empiric. Its major benefit appears to be in treating perianal disease, usually as an adjunct to corticosteroids. The response to metronidazole 1–2 g per day (15–20 $mg\,kg^{-1}\,day^{-1}$) may be gradual, with prolonged or indefinite treatment necessary because of relapses with tapering. Many clinicians are reluctant to use metronidazole in the long term because of its side-effects, especially peripheral neuropathy. More recently, ciprofloxacin 500 mg b.i.d. has been used as an alternative, based again primarily on empiric studies. The combination of metronidazole and ciprofloxacin may also be effective in some patients with refractory Crohn's disease, particularly those with fistulous disease.

Surgery

Surgery in Crohn's disease does not result in cure and is restricted to managing the complications of the disease or to disease not responsive to intensive medical therapy. About 80% of patients with Crohn's disease will require one or more operations. The intent of surgery should be conservative with preservation of bowel.

Postoperative recurrence remains a problem, with endoscopic recurrence occurring in 80–90% of patients

Notes

within 1 year and clinical recurrence occurring in up to 85% within 3 years. Recent evidence suggests that mesalazine (1.5–3 g per day, commencing within 1 month of surgery) can significantly reduce the frequency and severity of endoscopic recurrence, and possibly the rate of clinical recurrence, after ileocolonic resection.

Nutritional support

Enteric tube feeding with elemental, semielemental, or polymeric liquid diets has been studied as primary therapy for active Crohn's disease. Elemental formulae appear to offer no advantage over nonelemental formulae. Although liquid diet therapy may assist in remission induction in Crohn's disease, it is no more effective than corticosteroids. Neither enteral nor parenteral feeding is effective as primary therapy in active ulcerative colitis. Thus, the prime role of nutritional therapy in inflammatory bowel disease is adjunctive.

Nutritional deficiencies should be identified and replaced. If mild to moderate malnutrition is present then oral intake can be supplemented by encouraging a greater oral intake or by adding caloric supplements or a polymeric diet. If there is severe malnutrition, or oral intake is not expected for 3–5 days in a significantly malnourished patient, or oral intake is not expected for 5–8 days in a previously well nourished patient, then enteral tube, or possibly parenteral, nutritional supplementation is appropriate. Enteral feeding is preferred because it has significant advantages over parenteral feeding. The only absolute contraindication to enteral feeding is mechanical obstruction. Severe diarrhoea,

Notes

enteric fistulae, or a very short gut may provide special challenges to enteral feeding, but are not necessarily contraindications. Occasionally enteral feeds may need to be supplemented with parenteral nutrition.

The occurrence of lactose intolerance, previously thought to be common in inflammatory bowel disease, probably reflects underlying racial prevalence. It is also disputed that transient lactose intolerance may be associated with acute disease. Because of the importance of lactose-containing food products, lactase deficiency should be documented before any restriction (see *1.4.9 Overview of Malabsorption*).

In patients without active disease in whom there is mild diarrhoea due to impaired colonic water absorption, as may occur after ileocolonic resection or in quiescent pancolitis, antidiarrhoeals such as loperamide or diphenoxylate with atropine may be of benefit (see *2.2.1 Antidiarrhoeals*). These drugs should be avoided in active disease because of the risk of precipitating toxic megacolon. Diarrhoea in patients with nonobstructive ileal disease, or after ileocolonic resection, may be caused by excessive bile salts reaching the colonic lumen. This can usually be controlled by judicious use of cholestyramine.

1.4.22.3

PREGNANCY AND INFLAMMATORY BOWEL DISEASE

Fertility in women with ulcerative colitis appears not to be reduced. An exception may be patients with chronic active disease. In Crohn's disease, however, fertility in

Notes

women is often impaired. In men, *sulphasalazine* is the commonest cause of subfertility because of its effect on sperm (see *2.2.5 Sulphasalazine* and *2.2.6 Aminosalicylates*).

In ulcerative colitis, active disease at the start of the pregnancy usually continues, although severe deterioration is rare with current medications. However, the more difficult it is to control the active disease the lower is the chance of a normal live birth. If ulcerative colitis is in remission at the start of pregnancy, relapse occurs in about one third of patients, similar to the rate in nonpregnant women. Relapse is most common in the first trimester. In successive pregnancies the course of disease is usually unpredictable, although consistent deterioration may occur in a small proportion of patients (about 15%). The first attack of ulcerative colitis can occur during pregnancy (usually in the first trimester) or in the puerperium. In early series, this ran a severe course in about half of the patients, with a high maternal mortality rate (about 15%). This has not been the case in more recent studies.

In Crohn's disease, disease in remission at the start of pregnancy relapses infrequently (approximately 15%). If a relapse occurs it is usually in the first trimester or puerperium. If the disease is active at the beginning of pregnancy it tends to improve in about one third of patients, to remain the same in one third, and to deteriorate in one third. In active Crohn's disease there is an increased risk of spontaneous abortion, prematurity, or stillbirth.

Investigation of active disease during pregnancy is similar to that noted above (see *Investigations, Ulcerative Colitis* or *Crohn's Disease* above), with the exception that radiologic investigations are usually avoided, especially

Notes

in the first trimester. Radiography may sometimes be necessary, however, in the management of severely ill patients.

Medical or surgical treatment of inflammatory bowel disease during pregnancy is similar to that in the nonpregnant patient. Neither sulphasalazine nor corticosteroids have an adverse effect on the chance of having a normal child. Overall disease activity is the most important predictor of foetal outcome. The newer salicylates, however, are not recommended during pregnancy because experience is limited. Continued use of azathioprine during pregnancy is probably safe, although experience is limited. As such, most clinicians attempt to cease azathioprine before conception; however, it is important to maintain remission. Other second-line therapies are probably best avoided.

After resection for inflammatory bowel disease, including colectomy with ileostomy or ileoanal pouch, there is a good chance of a normal outcome in any subsequent pregnancy.

1.4.23

Watery Diarrhoea–Colitis Syndrome (Collagenous and Lymphocytic Microscopic Colitis)

The term watery diarrhoea–colitis syndrome (WDCS) encompasses the condition in a group of patients who have histologic evidence of colitis but a normal or near-normal macroscopic appearance of the colonic mucosa,

Notes

and in whom there is idiopathic watery diarrhoea. Histologically biopsies may show a thickened collagenous band (mean 10–30 μm) beneath the subepithelial membrane; termed *collagenous colitis*. Alternatively, the biopsies may demonstrate a mild to moderate increase in chronic and acute inflammatory cells in the lamina propria associated with a marked increase in intraepithelial lymphocytes; termed *lymphocytic colitis* or *microscopic colitis*. These histologic appearances may vary in intensity, and biopsies from around the colon may be necessary for diagnosis.

EPIDEMIOLOGY AND PATHOGENESIS

Collagenous colitis and lymphocytic microscopic colitis have become increasingly recognized over the past 10–15 years with the growing use of colonoscopy and mucosal biopsy in the investigation of diarrhoea. They account for about 1–2% of patients who undergo colorectal biopsy for nonneoplastic conditions.

The peak time of presentation is the sixth decade and approximately 80% of reported cases have been in women. However, childhood cases and familial clustering have been documented. There are reported associations with a variety of extraintestinal disorders. These include thyroid disease, rheumatoid arthritis, and seronegative arthritis.

Lymphocytic microscopic colitis and collagenous colitis, although clinically similar, are probably distinct entities. Most cases reported initially as lymphocytic microscopic colitis do not subsequently develop a thickened subepithelial collagenous band. The apparent

Notes

development of a collagenous band in some patients with lymphocytic microscopic colitis may be due to inadequate initial sampling and misclassification.

The colitis is responsible for and not the result of the chronic diarrhoea. In collagenous colitis, perfusion studies have demonstrated active secretion of chloride ions into the colonic lumen with passive transfer of sodium and water. Colonic fluid absorption is also severely depressed in lymphocytic microscopic colitis.

PRESENTATION

Patients with WDCS present with a chronic history of watery, nonbloody diarrhoea that is usually intermittent but may be persistent. The diarrhoea may be large in volume with up to 20 stools per day. There may be associated abdominal pain, distension, weight loss, anorexia, flatulence, and nausea.

INVESTIGATIONS

Stool microscopy and culture are normal. Faecal osmolarity suggests a secretory diarrhoea. Tests for small bowel malabsorption or maldigestion are normal; an exception is the rare association with probable coeliac disease. Imaging of the small and large bowel is usually normal. Abnormal colonic biopsies are critical for the diagnosis.

MANAGEMENT

Although there have been no controlled therapeutic trials, rapid clinical improvement is usually achieved

Notes

with oral *corticosteroids,* starting at a high dose and tapering over 4–6 weeks. Subsequent remission is usually sustained for prolonged periods of time, in some patients for years. Other conventional drugs for inflammatory bowel disease such as *sulphasalazine,* metronidazole, and local *corticosteroids,* although reported to be of benefit, are probably less effective than oral corticosteroids. There may also be symptomatic improvement with antidiarrhoeal drugs.

Liver and Biliary Disease

1.5.1

Variceal Bleeding

Variceal bleeding and ascites are direct consequences of portal hypertension. In patients with cirrhosis, bleeding varices account, primarily, for the high associated mortality rate.

EPIDEMIOLOGY AND PATHOGENESIS

Portal hypertension develops initially from an increase in resistance to portal flow, which follows the distortion of the liver microcirculation which is secondary to scarring, compression, and narrowing of the hepatic sinusoids. Portal hypertension can also occur where there is blockage of the portal vein (prehepatic) or as a result of blockage in the hepatic venous system (posthepatic).

Normal portal pressure is 5–8 mmHg, but as the portal pressure rises above 10–12 mmHg the venous system dilates and portosystemic collaterals develop in an attempt to decompress and reduce portal pressure. The main sites for collaterals are at the gastrooesophageal junction, the rectum, the left renal vein, the diaphragm, the retroperitoneum, and on the anterior abdominal wall via the umbilical vein. The collaterals shunt large amounts of portal blood away from the liver inducing detrimental hepatic and metabolic effects and causing the gastrooesophageal collaterals to dilate to form gastrooesophageal varices.

Variceal haemorrhage can occur if the portal pressure is greater than 12 mmHg, and although 75% of cirrhotics develop varices only 30% ever bleed. The risk of recurrent variceal haemorrhage after control of the initial

Notes

bleeding episode can be as high as 70% (Childs–Pugh cirrhosis grade C), and the 30-day mortality rate approaches 40% (grade C). The chance of bleeding is increased by large varices with a high portal pressure in patients with more severe liver dysfunction (*Figure 4*).

PRESENTATION

Haematemesis and melena is the usual mode of presentation, although occult bleeding can rarely occur. The bleeding may be torrential and can precipitate hepatic encephalopathy. Some 20% die during the first episode of bleeding. Bleeding that passed unnoticed can be the precipitating factor in patients presenting with decompensated cirrhosis (encephalopathy and/or ascites).

MANAGEMENT

Initial therapy is aimed at correcting hypovolemic shock and achieving haemostasis at the bleeding site (*Figure*

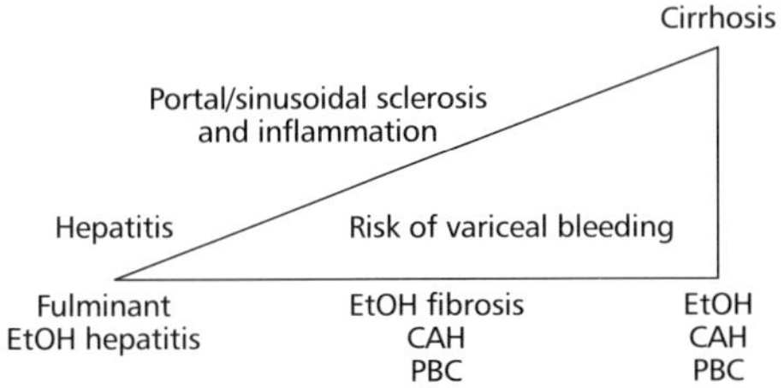

Figure 4 Risk of bleeding in intrahepatic portal hypertension. EtOH, alcohol or alcohol-related; CAH, chronic active hepatitis; PBC, primary biliary cirrhosis.

Notes

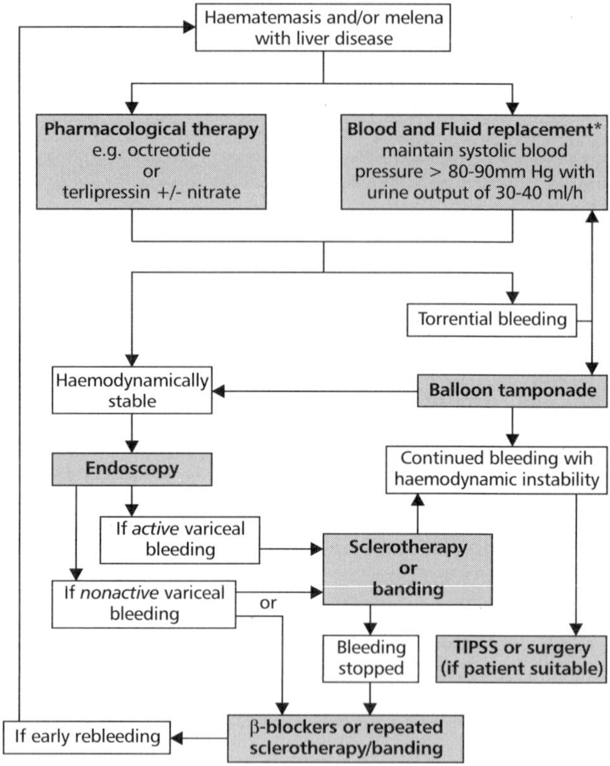

Figure 5 An approach to variceal bleeding. *Excessive volume replacement may be associated with rebound portal hypertension.

1.5

Notes

5). The general principles are the same as for other causes of upper gastrointestinal bleeding (see *1.3.2.1*). As patients with cirrhosis may bleed from sites other than gastrooesophageal varices (about 30%), emergency endoscopy should be one of the first steps. In unconscious patients endotracheal intubation should be used to avoid aspiration. If bleeding varices are found at endoscopy, an attempt should be made to control bleeding by endoscopic banding or sclerotherapy. If haemostasis is achieved, further banding or sclerotherapy is performed over the next few weeks. An alternative approach after initial control is the use of β-blockers (see below).

If initial endoscopic therapy is unsuccessful, and if rebleeding occurs, other measures are required. Balloon tamponade may be employed but it is associated with a high morbidity rate and the inflated balloons can be left in place only for up to 24 hours, but it is an effective holding procedure. Balloons inflated for longer periods cause ischemic mucosal ulceration.

Emergency surgery is used when sclerotherapy fails to control the bleeding, particularly if the bleeding is from gastric fundal varices. Oesophageal transection is the most usual operation performed, although portosystemic shunt surgery is still employed in the United States. Gastric devascularization is sometimes another option. Transjugular intrahepatic portal–systemic shunting (TIPSS) is successfully used in specialized centers as a method of decompressing the portal system without requiring abdominal surgery.

There are several pharmacologic treatments available that may control variceal bleeding. Drugs are aimed at

Notes

arresting variceal haemorrhage by decreasing pressure and blood flow in the oesophageal varices. The main groups of drugs used are vasopressin or analogues (terlipressin) and somatostatin or analogues (*octreotide*). If there is a strong suspicion at presentation that bleeding is variceal then one of these drugs should be started immediately. Otherwise the tendency is to await endoscopic confirmation before commencement.

Vasopressin is administered as a continuous intravenous. infusion starting at 0.4 units per min and increased, if necessary, to 0.6 and 0.8 units per min. Therapy is usually maintained until bleeding has been controlled for 12–24 hours. If more than 0.4 units per min are required, the rate of infusion is decreased stepwise before stopping treatment. Vasopressin use is limited by many side-effects due to systemic vasoconstriction and cardiotoxicity. These effects can be minimized by using glyceryl trinitrate either sublingually, intravenously, or transdermally (10 mg per 24 hours), and the use of nitrates should be considered in all patients with a history of ischaemic heart disease. Patients given vasopressin invariably complain of colicky abdominal pain and have a marked facial pallor owing to the generalized vasoconstriction.

The synthetic analogue of vasopressin, terlipressin, can be used in intravenous injections of 2 mg every 4 hours. It has the advantage that bolus injections can be used as it slowly releases vasopressin after intravenous bolus injection. It is likely, although unproven, that terlipressin has fewer side-effects than vasopressin, and it has been shown to reduce mortality. As with vasopressin, terlipressin is often coadministered with a nitrate.

Notes

As an alternative, somatostatin or its long-acting analogue, octreotide can be administered for 3–5 days. Somatostatin is given as a 250-μg bolus dose followed by an infusion of 250 μg per hour. Octreotide is given as a 50 μg bolus dose followed by an infusion of 50 μg per hour. These drugs produce an initial vasoconstriction without significant systemic vascular effects or complications. They are at least as effective as vasopressin or terlipressin in the control of acute bleeding.

Prevention of rebleeding

Recurrent banding or sclerotherapy after the first variceal bleed reduces rebleeding, and also reduces mortality. Recurrent banding, but not sclerotherapy, may also be beneficial as primary prophylaxis in preventing bleeding and reducing mortality in patients with large varices.

Pharmacologic prophylaxis of variceal rebleeding with the β-blocker propranolol is as effective as sclerotherapy. Combination of β-blockers with sclerotherapy, however, does not confer any additional advantage. The dose of propranolol should be high enough to reduce the heart rate by 25% or to reduce hepatic vein pressure by 25% or to a level less than 12 mmHg. However, there are nonresponders to propranolol in terms of portal pressure reduction. Some patients may also tolerate the medication poorly.

Propranolol is also effective when used as primary prophylaxis in patients at higher risk of bleeding, defined by the presence of large varices, or varices with a hepatic venous pressure greater than 12 mmHg. Thus at first diagnosis of cirrhosis, endoscopic assessment for varices

Notes

should be considered. If β-blockers are not initiated, subsequent endoscopic monitoring at 1–2-year intervals is probably appropriate.

Portosystemic shunts, oesophageal transection, devascularization procedures, and transplantation all remain options if rebleeding episodes cannot be prevented. With the exception of transplantation, none is associated with improved survival because of the commensurate increase in death from hepatic failure.

1.5.2

Ascites

Ascites is defined as free fluid in the peritoneal space. Approximately 500 ml of fluid needs to be present before it is detectable clinically by percussion, although smaller amounts can be shown by abdominal ultrasonography. Twenty-five litres of fluid may be present in some patients with "tense" ascites.

There are many causes of ascites (*Table 26*). A serum : ascites albumin ratio greater than 1.1 is highly suggestive of a transudate. A difference of 11 $g\,l^{-1}$ between the serum albumin and the ascites albumin concentration is diagnostic of a transudate secondary to portal hypertension.

Chylous ascites is rare and occurs when there is obstruction to the thoracic duct preventing lymphatic outflow from the abdomen. The diagnosis of chylous ascites is suspected when milky fluid is obtained on a diagnostic tap and confirmed by the presence of high concentrations of triglyceride (greater than 200 $mg\,dl^{-1}$) in the fluid.

Notes

Table 26 Common causes of ascites

Transudate*	Exudate†
Parenchymal liver disease (e.g. cirrhosis)	Peritoneal metastases
Right ventricular failure	Pancreatitis (acute or chronic)
Constrictive pericarditis	Peritonitis (bacteria or tuberculosis)
Portal vein occlusion	Ovarian tumour (Meigs' syndrome)
Budd–Chiari syndrome	Chylous

* *Ascitic protein level* $< 25\ g\ l^{-1}$; *serum albumin minus ascites albumin* $> 11\ g\ l^{-1}$.

† *Ascitic protein level* $> 25\ g\ l^{-1}$; *serum albumin minus ascites albumin* $< 11\ g\ l^{-1}$.

1.5.2.1

HEPATIC ASCITES

EPIDEMIOLOGY AND PATHOGENESIS

Over 60% of cirrhotics develop ascites at some stage. The occurrence of ascites carries a poor prognosis with 25–50% of patients not surviving 1 year.

The pathophysiology of ascites formation in cirrhosis is complex and incompletely understood. Hepatic factors include changes in hepatic and intestinal lymph formation, low serum albumin levels, increases in hepatic sinusoidal pressure, and consequent increase in portal vein pressure. In addition, changes in renal function, particularly renal sodium handling, have to be considered.

One hypothesis, the "overflow theory", suggests that the primary event is renal retention of sodium leading to

Notes

plasma volume expansion. With increased hepatic lymph production, increase of the hepatic sinusoidal vein pressure and lowered oncotic pressure, fluid becomes localized in the peritoneal cavity.

An alternative theory, "underfill", suggests that blood pools in the splanchnic circulation. In addition, the excess lymph weeps into the peritoneal cavity which in combination with a lowered systemic vascular resistance causes a decreased effective plasma volume. The low effective blood volume stimulates the sympathetic nervous system, activates the renin–angiotensin–aldosterone system, and results in increased renal sodium and water retention. Decreased secretion of renal prostaglandins and vasoactive substances can lead to severe functional renal failure with reduced glomerular filtration.

These concepts are not mutually exclusive and overflow may be followed by underfill (see *Figure 6*).

PRESENTATION

Clinical history and examination often indicates the cause of ascites. Signs of chronic liver disease and cardiac causes should be sought. Evaluation of the jugular venous pressure is important. A massive ovarian cyst may be mistaken for ascites.

INVESTIGATIONS

Ultrasonography is especially useful in excluding primary and secondary hepatic tumours and in providing information on vascular causes such as Budd–Chiari syndrome. A 10–20-ml aspirate of ascites, a

Notes

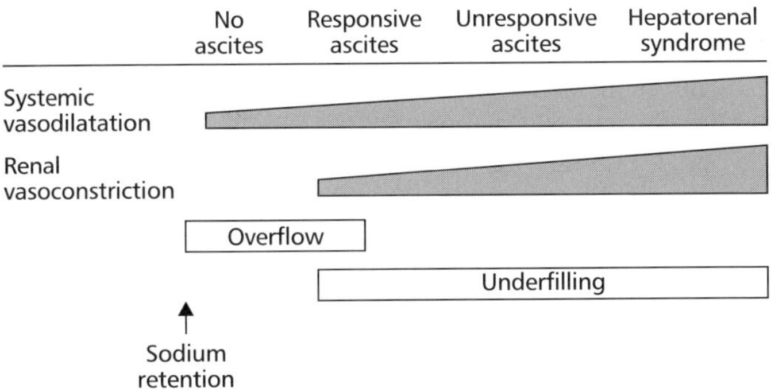

Figure 6 Schematic representation of the relationship between renal sodium retention and changes in systemic and renal haemodynamics at various stages of cirrhosis. Adapted from Wong F and Blendis L. *Seminars in Liver Disease* 1994; **14**: 2 (with permission).

"diagnostic tap", is mandatory for microscopy and culture, cytology, albumin, and total protein estimation (see *1.5.3 Spontaneous Bacterial Peritonitis*). Other laboratory tests on ascitic fluid that may be helpful are amylase (raised in pancreatitis and gut perforation), bilirubin if ascitic fluid is bile stained (ascitic fluid bilirubin: serum bilirubin > 1.0 – biliary perforation), and triglycerides if ascitic fluid is opalescent or frankly milky.

MANAGEMENT

Patients developing moderate or tense ascites should be admitted to hospital. Dietary sodium is reduced to 50 mmol per day (normal 100–150 mmol per day) initially

Notes

and, in severe cases, to 22 mmol per day; fluids are restricted to 1500 ml daily. Bedrest should be reserved for patients with tense ascites. These measures alone will frequently result in a diuresis and mobilization of the ascitic fluid in mild cases, although the majority of patients require diuretic therapy. Distal potassium-sparing diuretics should be used as first-line agents; oral spironolactone (100 mg initially) is normally chosen. It normally takes 24–48 hours before effective diuresis occurs. Amiloride (5–20 mg per day) is an alternative, but is probably not as effective as spironolactone. Loop diuretics (frusemide, bumetanide) are not very effective without a distal nephron diuretic (spironolactone).

There are two diuretic schedules that are usually used in hepatic ascites: (1) increasing doses (every 3 days) of spironolactone (100-mg increments to 400–600 mg per day), adding frusemide only to those patients not responding to the higher doses of spironolactone; or (2) simultaneous administration of spironolactone and frusemide from the beginning with increasing doses of both diuretics (i.e. 100 mg/40 mg, 200 mg/80 mg, 300 mg/120 mg, 400 mg/160 mg) until a therapeutic response is achieved. The second regimen is most suited to non-azotemic patients with severe ascites. A weight loss of approximately 0.5 kg daily should be aimed at; in patients without peripheral oedema greater diuresis can reduce plasma volume and precipitate renal failure and encephalopathy. Patients with peripheral oedema are at less risk of plasma volume depletion and a weight loss of up to 1.5 kg per day can be achieved safely in these patients. Signs of encephalopathy, postural hypotension, renal failure, and electrolyte disturbance should be sought.

Notes

Abdominal paracentesis of 5 litres per day, or draining to dryness with intravenous albumin replacement (6–8 $g\,l^{-1}$ of ascites removed), has been shown to be as effective as diuretic therapy without adverse side-effects in patients with stable hepatic function. This procedure can also be employed in refractory cases. A permanent peritoneal–venous shunt (Le-Veen shunt) can also be tried in patients with refractory ascites, although there is a high risk of infection and disseminated intravascular coagulation. TIPSS (transjugular intrahepatic portal–systemic shunting) can also be successful in the treatment of refractory ascites.

Patients receiving diuretic therapy may develop prerenal failure, often associated with hyponatremia. Diuretic therapy should be stopped and strict fluid restriction of 800 ml to 1 litre per day should be enforced.

In patients with severe liver disease, who are often deeply jaundiced, functional renal failure (hepatorenal syndrome) can develop with or without acute tubular necrosis. It is characterized by a very low urinary sodium concentration. Initial treatment consists of maintenance of intravascular pressures with colloid, but the prognosis is very poor. Dopamine infusion (2–4 $\mu g\,kg^{-1}$ per hour) may help, but can be deleterious when tachycardia is present.

1.5.3

Spontaneous Bacterial Peritonitis

Spontaneous bacterial peritonitis (SBP) is defined as bacterial infection of ascitic fluid without any intra-abdominal source of infection.

Notes

EPIDEMIOLOGY AND PATHOGENESIS

Spontaneous bacterial peritonitis is a frequent and severe complication of cirrhotic patients with ascites. The incidence of SBP in patients admitted to hospital with ascites ranges from 7 to 23%. The probability of recurrence of SBP within 1 year is about 70%. The hospital mortality rate of cirrhotics with SBP is 30–50%, compared with more than 80% before 1980. This reduced mortality is due to increased awareness, early diagnosis, and more appropriate treatment.

The majority of SBP is caused by microorganisms of intestinal origin, particularly enterobacteria, and is nearly always monomicrobial (92%). The pathogenesis of SBP involves transportation of gut bacteria across the gut mucosa to mesenteric lymphatics and contamination of blood by culture-positive lymph. Prolonged bacteremia as a result of complement deficiency, neutrophil dysfunction and reticuloendothelial dysfunction also plays a part. Seeding of ascitic fluid with bloodborne bacteremia and lastly uncontrolled growth of bacteria in opsonin-deficient ascites is important.

PRESENTATION

The majority of patients with SBP have signs of systemic infection, although less than 50% of patients have abdominal pain or tenderness. Localizing signs are frequently absent. Because specific signs of SBP may be absent in a significant proportion of patients, diagnostic paracentesis should be performed routinely in any patient presenting with ascites and whenever hepatic

Notes

encephalopathy, progressive renal failure, or gastrointestinal haemorrhage occur.

INVESTIGATION

A diagnostic abdominal paracentesis is the key investigation. Analysis of the fluid is mandatory before a diagnosis of SBP can be established. The ascitic neutrophil count is the single best predictor of SBP and can be estimated rapidly. A neutrophil count of greater than 250 cells per mm^3 (0.25×10^9 cells per litre) is strong evidence of SBP infection, and greater than 500 cells per mm^3 is diagnostic. Ascitic culture is helpful and maximal yield is obtained by inoculating blood culture bottles with ascitic fluid at the bedside. Blood cultures should also be taken as they are positive in about 50% of ascitic fluid culture-positive SBP episodes and 33% of culture-negative SBP episodes.

About 70% of cases are caused by aerobic Gram-negative bacilli, especially *Escherichia coli* and *Klebsiella*. In the remainder, aerobic Gram-positive cocci are usually responsible, especially *Streptococcus* species (*S. pneumoniae*). Anaerobes are an infrequent cause because of the high partial pressure of oxygen of ascites. Fungi do not cause SBP.

Other laboratory tests on ascitic fluid that may be helpful are total protein, albumin, amylase, Gram stain, cytology, and triglycerides (see *1.5.2.1 Hepatic Ascites*).

MANAGEMENT

As soon as the diagnosis is established, treatment should be started with a third-generation cephalosporin, such as

Notes

cefotaxime 2 g intravenously every 8 hours. An alternative is intravenous amoxycillin–clavulanic acid. If there is significant allergy to β-lactams then vancomycin or clindamycin, combined with either aztreonam or a quinilone or aminoglycoside, is a suitable empiric regimen. Treatment should be for 5 days in the first instance and may need to be tailored according to the responsible pathogen. Repeat ascitic tap can be performed in 2–3 days to confirm response.

Primary prophylaxis by selective intestinal decontamination should be considered in patients with ascites who are at high risk of developing SBP. Such high-risk patients include those with a low ascitic total protein level ($<1\ \mathrm{g\,dl^{-1}}$), increased bilirubin level ($> 2.5\ \mathrm{mg\,dl^{-1}}$), gastrointestinal haemorrhage, and acute liver failure. Prophylaxis after one episode of SBP as been shown to reduce the likelihood of further recurrence. *Norfloxacin* (400 mg orally daily) or *ciprofloxacin* (750 mg orally once per week) has been shown to be effective for both primary and secondary prophylaxis.

1.5.4

Hepatic Encephalopathy

The term hepatic encephalopathy is applied to a spectrum of neuropsychiatric syndromes that may develop in liver disease. The most common type of hepatic encephalopathy is portosystemic encephalopathy (PSE) which occurs almost exclusively in patients with cirrhosis with portal hypertension and portosystemic shunting. In these patients there may be

Notes

no obvious precipitating factor, apart from excess dietary protein, and the hepatocellular disease may be relatively stable. More rarely chronic neuropsychiatric states exist, usually in patients with chronic portosystemic shunting, and are associated with irreversible brain damage.

EPIDEMIOLOGY AND PATHOGENESIS

The main types of hepatic encephalopathy are shown in *Table 27*. The outcome depends on the severity of the underlying liver damage.

Table 27 Main types of hepatic encephalopathy

Type	Episode survival (%)	Common causes
Acute or acute on chronic portosystemic (underlying cirrhosis)	70–80	Gastrointestinal haemorrhage Over-diuresis Dehydration Drugs, such as opiates Electrolyte disturbance Hypoglycemia General anaesthesia
Chronic portosystemic	**100**	Excess dietary protein Constipation Portocaval shunt
Acute liver failure	**20–30**	Viral hepatitis (all types) Drug reaction
Toxins		Wilson's disease

Notes

1.5

The diffuse nature of the cerebral dysfunction associated with hepatic encephalopathy, and the fact that it is potentially reversible, suggests that the cerebral change is metabolic in nature. Toxic metabolites produced in the gut, bypass the liver via the collateral portosystemic circulation, and then pass directly to the brain to produce the encephalopathy. Circumstantial evidence suggests that the toxic metabolites are produced by the intestinal bacteria, particularly in the colon. Ammonia, aromatic amino acids, mercaptans, free fatty acids, and false neurotransmitters such as octopamine, have been implicated.

Current evidence suggests that the inhibitory neurotransmitter γ-aminobutyric acid (GABA) is involved. It is produced by bacterial action within the gut and concentrations are increased in the blood of patients with hepatic encephalopathy. There is a close relationship between the GABA binding sites in the brain and those for benzodiazepines; both compounds promote chloride conduction across the postsynaptic neuromembrane, inhibiting postsynaptic potentials. GABA and benzodiazepine receptor antagonists such as flumazenil have been shown temporarily to ameliorate hepatic encephalopathy.

PRESENTATION

The clinical features of hepatic encephalopathy are variable. With acute onset, with a precipitating factor, or due to acute hepatic failure, the patient becomes increasingly drowsy and comatose. The grading of coma is shown in *Table 28*.

Notes

Table 28 Grade of hepatic encephalopathy

Grade	Signs and symptoms
1	Confusion, mood alteration, psychometric defects
2	Drowsiness
3	Stuporous, but rousable and may obey simple commands. Slurred speech
4	Coma
5	Deep coma with no response to painful stimuli

In chronic portosystemic encephalopathy (PSE) the changes are fluctuant, but are characterized by personality change, intellectual deterioration, and disturbed consciousness, with a disorder of sleep rhythm. Speech is low and slurred, with a monotonous voice. Other signs include a coarse flapping tremour (asterixis). This is demonstrated by outstretching the hands and hyper–extending the wrists. Foetor hepaticus, a characteristic sweet smell, may be detectable on the breath. There is often a marked constructional apraxia, so that the patient cannot write or draw, for example, a five-pointed star. The Reitan Trail Making test may be used serially to assess progress; this tests the ability to join numbers with a pencil within a certain time. In later stages of hepatic encephalopathy, coma develops, often together with convulsions, hyperventilation, and pyrexia.

INVESTIGATIONS

Investigations may be useful in selected patients. These include electroencephalography (EEG), which demon-

Notes

strates slowing of the frequency of the normal α range 8 to 13 cycles per second (c.p.s.) down to the δ range of below 4 c.p.s. These changes are not specific for liver disease and may also be found in uraemia and in carbon dioxide retention.

Measurement of the visually evoked potential gives an expression of postsynaptic cellular potential activity; it is a useful method for estimating the degree of encephalopathy and may predict those at risk. Patients in hepatic failure may show increased level of cerebrospinal fluid protein on lumbar puncture but the cell count is normal. Ammonia levels vary with severity, but 10% of values are in the normal range, regardless of the depth of coma. Serum ammonia levels may be useful if the cause of the coma is in doubt. Cranial computed tomography and magnetic resonance imaging has a role in selected patients; cerebral atrophy may be demonstrated particularly in patients with chronic PSE and a history of prolonged alcohol intake.

MANAGEMENT

The principles of treatment of hepatic encephalopathy are outlined in *Table 29*. One of the most effective measures is the use of *nonabsorbed carbohydrates* such as lactulose or lactitol (see *2.2.4.6 Hyperosmotic Laxatives*). These lower faecal pH, which enhances faecal ammonia excretion because of luminal trapping of ammonia as NH_4^+. If oral administration is undesirable or the patient is comatose, then lactulose enemas (500 ml plus 500 ml water) are effective. The production of ammonia by bacterial flora can be suppressed by the oral adminis-

Notes

Table 29 Treatment of hepatic encephalopathy

Acute	
1	Identify and treat precipitating cause (e.g. infection)
2	Empty bowels of nitrogen-containing material by use of magnesium sulphate or phosphate enema, then start lactulose 30 ml orally t.i.d. (see *2.2.4.6 Hyperosmotic Laxatives*)
3	Protein restriction to 20 g daily
4	Consider neomycin 1 g orally four times a day for 1 week
5	Stop or reduce diuretic therapy and correct electrolyte imbalances
6	Correct hypoglycemia
Chronic	
1	Allow protein intake to the limit of tolerance, usually about 60 g per day
2	Avoid constipation and ensure at least two free bowel movements per day by means of lactulose or lactitol (see *2.2.4.6*)
3	Avoid sedative drugs and over-diuresis

tration of a nonabsorbable antibiotic, such as neomycin. Long-term administration of neomycin, however, is undesirable because of potential side-effects such as deafness and renal tubular damage.

Although lactulose or lactitol given together with neomycin may have a synergistic effect on encephalopathy, they should be combined only if either is not producing optimal results. This is because in some patients they may diminish the effect of one another: neomycin activity is reduced by a reduced colonic pH,

Notes

and neomycin may prevent the degradation of lactulose. The functionality of the combination can be tested by measuring faecal pH, which should continue to be acidified (from 6.0–7.0 to 5.0–6.0) by lactulose.

1.5.5

Fulminant Hepatic Failure

Fulminant hepatic failure occurs when a previously normal liver fails acutely, resulting in a severe loss of hepatic function with encephalopathy. By definition, the encephalopathy develops within 8 weeks of the onset of first symptoms (especially jaundice) in a liver that has previously been normal.

EPIDEMIOLOGY AND PATHOGENESIS

Acute parenchymal liver damage (active hepatitis) is caused by a wide variety of agents (*Table 30*). The degree of hepatocellular damage for a given agent may be extremely variable, but impairment in the functions of the liver can result from generalized necrosis of hepatocytes. Overwhelming hepatocyte death may result in collapse of normal liver architecture and the development of fulminant hepatic failure.

It is important to attempt to ascertain the cause of the liver failure as the prognosis is strongly dependent on the etiology; for example 60% of patients with grade III coma will survive paracetamol overdose compared with only 20–30% of those with viral hepatitis. Elderly patients aged over 60 years also have a poor prognosis.

Notes

Table 30 Causes of acute parenchymal liver damage

Viral infections	
	Hepatotropic viruses (A, B, C, D, E)
	Nonhepatotropic viruses (e.g. cytomegalovirus, Epstein–Barr, herpes simplex)
Drugs	
	e.g. paracetamol, diclofenac
Poisons	
	e.g. *Amanita phalloides* (mushroom), carbon tetrachloride
Nonviral infections	
	e.g. leptospirosis, toxoplasmosis
Vascular	
	Prolonged hypotension, veno-occlusive disease, heat stroke, malignant infiltration
Miscellaneous	
	Reye's syndrome, acute fatty liver of pregnancy

PRESENTATION

Physical examination reveals a patient with jaundice with evidence of hepatic encephalopathy. Signs of chronic liver disease are usually absent, although palmar erythema and spider nevi can develop within 1 week to 10 days of the development of acute hepatic failure. Ascites and oedema may occur, although splenomegaly is uncommon. The liver is usually small, although hepatomegaly is found with some rarer causes.

The severity of the encephalopathy may fluctuate especially in the early phases. In more severe encephalo-

Notes

pathy there is a high risk of cerebral oedema (about 80% in patients with grade 4 encephalopathy). This may occur rapidly and is one of the major causes of death. Clinical signs associated with cerebral oedema include systemic hypertension, hyperventilation, abnormal papillary reflexes, papilledema, decerebrate posturing, and eventually impairment of brainstem reflexes and functions. Initially these signs may be paroxysmal and precipitated by tactile stimuli. Subsequently they become sustained.

INVESTIGATIONS

The most useful marker of the severity of the liver necrosis is the prothrombin time. Serum biochemistry reveals high levels of transaminases and bilirubin, which are not useful indicators of the prognosis. Serum albumin concentration is usually normal in the acute stages of the disease, but may fall over some weeks.

MANAGEMENT

All patients with fulminant hepatic failure should be admitted to an intensive care unit. Monitoring followed by supportive therapy is the mainstay of treatment. Severe acidosis ($pH < 7.3$) should be corrected and acid–base balance monitored regularly. Electrolyte balance should be maintained and intravenous potassium phosphate given if severe hypophosphatemia is present. Intravenous dextrose (10%) is given to prevent hypoglycemia, and blood glucose should be monitored regularly. *H_2-receptor antagonists* are given intravenously to reduce

Notes

the risk of gastrointestinal haemorrhage. If active bleeding occurs, fresh frozen plasma is given (vitamin K appears to be of little value) and platelets are infused if the platelet count is 50 000 per ml or less.

Encephalopathy is managed as described for hepatic encephalopathy (see *1.5.4*). Encephalopathy that does not progress beyond grade 2, irrespective of the cause, tends to have a good prognosis. Once grade 3 or 4 encephalopathy develops, however, there is a substantially increased risk of other complications (see *Table 31*) and outcome is less predictable.

The comatose patient is at high risk of cerebral oedema, and should be nursed in a quiet environment with minimal tactile stimulation, and positioned with the trunk and head elevated approximately 45° from the horizontal. In some institutions intracranial pressure monitoring is undertaken, although its use is controversial. Treatment of cerebral oedema is with mannitol (bolus infusion of 0.5 $g\,kg^{-1}$) repeated every 4 hours as necessary. Renal failure makes mannitol infusions ineffective and dangerous and may indicate a need for haemofiltration or haemodialysis.

Table 31 Complications of fulminant hepatic failure

Cerebral oedema
Renal failure
Gastrointestinal bleeding
Bacterial infection
Hypoglycemia
Spontaneous hypotension
Respiratory failure and respiratory arrest
Acute pancreatitis

Notes

When mannitol is ineffective or contraindicated, intravenous sodium thiopentone (1.5–3.5 $mg\,kg^{-1}$, intermittent boluses) may be effective if adequate ventilation is provided.

Renal failure, in the presence of adequate intravascular pressure, occurs in about 30% of patients with non-paracetamol fulminant hepatic failure and is usually associated with severe encephalopathy. In these patients it is due primarily to the development of hepatorenal syndrome with or without acute tubular necrosis. Renal failure is more frequent in patients with paracetamol-induced fulminant hepatic failure (about 75%), probably because of direct renal toxicity, and usually precedes the development of severe encephalopathy. Initial treatment consists of maintenance of intravascular pressure with colloid. Dopamine infusion (2–4 $\mu g\,kg^{-1}$ per hour) may help, but can be deleterious when tachycardia is present. Haemofiltration or haemdialysis may be necessary.

In suspected paracetamol overdose liver injury can be reduced by *N*-acetylcysteine (adults: initially 150 $mg\,kg^{-1}$ in 200 ml 5% dextrose intravenously over 15 min; then, continuous infusion of 50 $mg\,kg^{-1}$ in 500 ml 5% dextrose over 4 hours, followed by 100 $mg\,kg^{-1}$ in 1 litre of 5% dextrose over 16 hours). Early administration is most effective, although benefit occurs up to 36 hours or possibly longer after overdose. *N*-acetylcysteine may also be beneficial in nonparacetamol fulminant hepatic failure, partly because of improved haemodynamics and improved oxygen delivery to body tissues.

Fulminant hepatic failure is associated with a high incidence of bacterial infection. Fungal sepsis may also be a problem. The therapeutic usefulness of prophylactic antibiotics, however, is still unproven. Tight surveillance is

Notes

indicated with daily cultures of all available specimens. Positive cultures should be treated with appropriate antibiotics. Antibiotics and antifungals should be strongly considered in patients in whom there is a halting or reversal of improvement as this is often due to sepsis.

In patients who continue to deteriorate, orthotopic liver transplantation should be considered. The criteria for transplantation, as adopted in King's College Hospital (O'Grady JG, Alexander GJM, Hayllar KM, Williams R. *Gastroenterology* 1989; **97**: 439–45) and used in many other institutions, are shown in *Table 32*.

Table 32 Criteria for liver transplantation in fulminant hepatic failure

Paracetamol (acetaminophen)

pH < 7.3 (irrespective of encephalopathy grade)

or

Prothrombin time $>$ 100 seconds and serum creatinine concentration $> 0.3\ \text{mmol l}^{-1}$ and grade 3 or 4 encephalopathy

Nonparacetamol (nonacetaminophen)

Prothrombin time $>$ 100 seconds or INR $>$ 6.7 (irrespective of encephalopathy grade)

or

Any three of the following variables (irrespective of encephalopathy grade):

- Age $<$ 10 or $>$ 40 years
- Jaundice for $>$ 7 days before encephalopathy
- Unfavourable etiology (nonA, nonB hepatitis, halothane hepatitis, or drug reaction)
- Prothrombin time $>$ 50 seconds or INR $>$ 4
- Serum bilirubin level $> 300\ \mu\text{mol l}^{-1}$

INR, international normalized ratio.

Notes

1.5.6

Chronic Hepatitis

Chronic hepatitis is defined as inflammation of the liver that persists for more than 6 months, evidenced by a persistent increase in the level of serum alanine (ALAT) and aspartate (ASAT) aminotransferases. This definition is arbitrary, but is based on the clinical observation that acute self-limiting viral hepatitis usually resolves within 6 months. However, aminotransferases may be increased in several conditions that are not associated with chronic hepatitis, and the definition depends on histologic assessment.

The common causes of aminotransferase increase that are not due to chronic hepatitis are alcohol abuse, obesity causing a fatty liver, diabetes mellitus, drug reactions, and thyroid disease, particularly thyrotoxicosis.

EPIDEMIOLOGY AND PATHOGENESIS

The causes of chronic hepatitis are shown in *Table 33*. Most cases are caused by viral infection, drugs, or autoimmune hepatitis. However, hepatitis A and hepatitis E never progress to chronic hepatitis.

PRESENTATION

Chronic hepatitis is often difficult to diagnose, because patients may be asymptomatic or have only minor symptoms of malaise and fatigue. However the life-threatening complications of advanced liver disease and hepatic failure can occur without warning. Most patients

Notes

Table 33 Main causes of chronic nonalcoholic liver disease

Diseases	Causes
Chronic hepatitis	Viral hepatitis Hepatitis B virus Hepatitis D (δ) virus Hepatitis C virus Autoimmune hepatitis Drug-induced hepatitis e.g. isoniazid, methyldopa, trielinic acid, nitrofurantoin, oxyphenisatin
Chronic metabolic liver disease	Nonalcoholic steatosis Idiopathic haemochromatosis Wilson's disease α_1-Antitrypsin deficiency
Chronic cholestatic syndromes	Primary biliary cirrhosis (PBC) Primary sclerosing cholangitis (PSC) Sarcoidosis Autoimmune cholangitis

who have raised serum levels of aminotransferases on routine biochemical screening are asymptomatic. Moreover, most of those who are not alcoholics will not have significant liver disease. However, because of the potentially serious consequences of missing chronic hepatitis in an early asymptomatic and treatable stage, all patients with persistently raised levels of aminotransferases need to be evaluated thoroughly.

INVESTIGATIONS

A full and careful history should be taken, with particular reference to alcohol consumption, previous

Notes

blood transfusions, recreational drug abuse and drugs, including over-the-counter remedies such as nonsteroidal anti-inflammatory drugs and herbal remedies. A complete physical examination, with particular reference to signs of chronic liver disease, should be performed. The screening investigations are shown in *Table 34*. An ultrasonographic examination of the liver and biliary tree should be performed to exclude structural lesions and to look for evidence of a fatty liver. If these noninvasive investigations are inconclusive, or suggest chronic hepatitis, the patient should be referred to a specialist

Table 34 Noninvasive investigations for chronic hepatitis

Full blood count and platelet count
Serum aminotransferases
Serum γ-glutamyl transpeptidase
Serum bilirubin
Serum alkaline phosphatase
Prothrombin time or ratio (INR)
Serology for hepatitis B and C
Serum autoantibodies, in particular:
Smooth muscle antibody (SMA)
Antinuclear factor (ANF)
Liver–kidney–microsomal antibody (LKM)
Antimitochondrial antibody (AMA)
Serum immunoglobulins
Serum iron, total iron-binding capacity, and transferrin saturation
Serum ceruloplasmin and copper; urinary 24 copper (in patients under 40 years)
Serum α_1-antitrypsin
Random blood alcohol
Thyroid function tests
Fasting blood sugar (if fatty liver on ultrasonography)

Notes

for further investigations, the first of which would be liver biopsy.

Hepatic histology may sometimes give the underlying cause of the chronic liver disease if hepatitis B or C antigens are found. However, the underlying cause of the chronic inflammation may not be apparent. A combination of the history, screening investigations, and histology is required to make a precise diagnosis.

Chronic hepatitis is classified into three types: chronic active hepatitis, chronic persistent hepatitis, and lobular hepatitis. Chronic active hepatitis is characterized by a chronic lymphocytic inflammatory infiltrate, which extends beyond the boundary of the portal tract into the hepatic lobule. In contrast, in chronic persistent hepatitis the portal lymphocytic infiltration is confined to the portal tract. In chronic lobular hepatitis there are areas of focal necrosis throughout the hepatic lobule, with or without inflammation of the portal triads.

In general, chronic active hepatitis is thought to be the most serious histologic abnormality, indicative of likely progression to bridging fibrosis and ultimately cirrhosis. However, it is clear that in some conditions, particularly hepatitis C, patients may progress to cirrhosis and hepatocellular carcinoma despite apparently innocuous liver histology.

MANAGEMENT

The decision to treat chronic hepatitis is made on the basis of symptoms, liver histology, and the underlying cause. This decision should always be made by a

Notes

specialist. Treatment of chronic hepatitis depends on the underlying cause and the histologic severity of the disease.

1.5.7

Overview of Viral Hepatitis

Many viruses are known to invade the liver. They are divided into (a) hepatotropic viruses that primarily reside and replicate in the liver; and (b) nonhepatotropic viruses in which the liver is involved as part of systemic infection (*Table 35*). Over the last decade, two or three new hepatotropic viruses have been identified (hepatitis C and E, and possibly hepatitis G). The features of the hepatotropic viruses are contrasted in *Table 36*. It is likely that several more viruses will be identified which cause hepatitis.

1.5.8

Hepatitis A (HAV Hepatitis)

EPIDEMIOLOGY AND PATHOGENESIS

The hepatitis A virus causes between 20 and 40% of clinically apparent cases of hepatitis. It occurs throughout the world and frequently causes epidemics which are seen most commonly in lower socioeconomic groups. In Western countries, attacks follow summer holidays in parts of the world where sanitation is poor and endemicity of hepatitis A is high. In northern European

Notes

Table 35 Viruses associated with hepatitis

Type of virus	Examples
Hepatotropic viruses	Hepatitis A Hepatitis B Hepatitis C Hepatitis D Hepatitis E (?Hepatitis G)
Nonhepatotropic viruses Systemic virosis in which hepatitis may be the main clinical picture	Cytomegalovirus (CMV) Epstein–Barr virus (EBV)
Nonhepatotropic viruses Systemic virosis occasionally producing hepatitis (especially in neonates or immunocompromised patients)	Herpes simplex virus Varicella zoster virus Rubeola (measles) virus Rubella (German measles) virus Coxsackie viruses Echoviruses Adenoviruses
Human immunodeficiency virus (HIV)	*All of the above viruses* are either more likely to occur or more likely to be associated with hepatic injury in patients with HIV infection

countries the disease is found in adults, although in areas where the hepatitis is endemic, children are usually affected at an early age.

Hepatitis A virus is a small (27 nm) RNA virus. The incubation period is usually 2–6 weeks, resulting in a

Notes

1.5

Table 36 The hepatitis viruses A–G contrasted

	A	B	C	D	E	G
Type	RNA	DNA	RNA	RNA	RNA	RNA
Size (nm)	27	42	30–60		27–32	30
Incubation period	2–6 weeks	1–6 months	2–8 weeks	1–6 months	2–9 weeks	Not known
Spread						
Blood	No	Yes	Yes	Yes	No	Yes
Feces	Yes	No	No	No	Yes	No
Saliva	Yes	Yes	?	Yes	No	Yes
Vertical	No	Yes	?No	Yes	No	Yes
Sexual	Uncommon	Yes	Yes	Yes	No	Yes
Treatment	Symptomatic	Symptomatic Interferon ?Antivirals	Symptomatic Interferon ?Antivirals	Symptomatic ?Antivirals	Symptomatic	Symptomatic
Prevention	Vaccine Immunoglobulin	Vaccine Immunoglobulin	None	Vaccine (hepatitis B)	None	None
Carrier state	No	Yes	Yes	Yes	No	Yes
Chronic hepatitis	No	10%	50–60%	50%	No	?
Liver cancer	No	Yes	Yes	No	No	?

Notes

variable prodromal illness before the onset of jaundice. HAV is secreted in the feces of infected persons for 2 weeks before the onset of the prodromal illness and for up to 7 days afterwards. Paradoxically, the excretion of virus in the stool drops dramatically at the onset of jaundice. The spread of infection is *mainly* by the faecal–oral route and arises from the ingestion of contaminated food or water. HAV infection may also be sexually transmitted in homosexual men.

PRESENTATION

The prodromal phase usually lasts up to 2 weeks before the onset of jaundice. During this time the patient feels generally unwell with nausea, vomiting, diarrhoea, and anorexia. A low-grade fever may occur together with right upper quadrant discomfort in the abdomen. With the onset of jaundice, the symptoms improve rapidly. Normally the jaundice settles after 2–4 weeks. A minority of patients will have a prolonged cholestatic jaundice lasting 6–16 weeks. Some patients will suffer a relapse. The relapse may last for several months but is usually associated with full recovery. Rarely fulminant hepatitis may develop which can progress to liver coma and death.

INVESTIGATIONS

Serum transaminase concentrations are raised, usually reaching peak levels (up to 3000 $IU\,l^{-1}$) 1–2 days before the development of jaundice. The transaminase levels usually then fall, but may remain increased for up to 6 months, sometime longer. Serum alkaline phosphatase

Notes

levels are usually less than three times the upper limit of normal. Serum bilirubin levels vary widely from patient to patient and may remain normal in anicteric hepatitis. Diagnosis is confirmed by the presence of antiHAV immunoglobulin (Ig) M antibody. IgG HAV antibodies are common in adult patients aged over 50 years and indicate a past infection. Liver biopsy is not routinely indicated, but should be performed when there is diagnostic uncertainty.

MANAGEMENT

There is no specific treatment. Conventionally patients are advised to take a low fat diet, rest, and avoid alcohol, but there is little evidence that this alters the course of the disease. Corticosteroids are indicated in only a few patients with prolonged cholestatic symptoms. Patients with dehydration because of persistent vomiting may require hospital admission. Otherwise, only patients with signs of liver failure are admitted.

The prognosis is good, with all patients who survive making a full recovery, as hepatitis A never progresses to chronic liver disease. The mortality rate in large epidemics is less than one per 10^5 and usually results from the development of fulminant hepatic necrosis.

Close personal contacts and patients without antiHAV antibodies travelling to endemic areas should be given immune serum globulin by intramuscular injection which offers protection for approximately 3 months. Sound hygiene and good sanitation are important for the prevention of epidemics.

An alternaytive for travellers to endemic areas is vaccination. A single dose of (Haruis 1440) gives protection, within two weeks of administration, lasting

Notes

up to 1 year, and boster at 6–12 months extends protection to at least 10 years.

1.5.9

Hepatitis B (HBV Hepatitis)

EPIDEMIOLOGY AND PATHOGENESIS

Hepatitis B is a major cause of disease worldwide. The population carriage rate of hepatitis B surface antigen (HBsAg) varies worldwide, from 0.1–0.2% in Britain and the United States to 10–15% in Africa and the Far East. Parenteral routes of infection include transfusion of infected blood or blood products, contaminated needles or syringes used by drug addicts and needlestick injuries. Hepatitis B virus is present in semen, saliva, and vaginal secretions, and can be transmitted by sexual intercourse, particularly in homosexuals. In high carriage rate areas, infection is often acquired by vertical transmission from mother to neonate during parturition.

Hepatitis B virus belongs to the hepadna viruses. The Dane particle, which consists of the whole virus, can be identified in the serum, an inner core comprises circular DNA and DNA polymerase, the core antigen and the e antigen, and an outer surface coat (HBsAg).

People who have acute HBV infection as an *adult* have a more than 90% chance of subsequently clearing the virus. About two thirds of acute HBV infections are subclinical. Fulminant acute hepatitis occurs rarely, but often has a fatal outcome (about 1%). However, if the patient survives a fulminant attack, recovery is complete without the development of chronic liver disease. About 5–10% of patients go on to develop chronic infection. The majority of those with chronic infection will remain asymptomatic

Notes

without any long-term sequelae; however, some will develop chronic hepatitis, cirrhosis and/or hepatoma.

Acquisition of HBV as an infant or child, which is most common in undeveloped areas of the world, is associated with about a 90% chance of chronic infection. These children have a lifetime risk of more than 25% of death from either cirrhosis or hepatocellular carcinoma.

There is a strong association between the prolonged carriage of HBV virus and development of primary liver cell cancer. Hepatocellular carcinoma is more common in men than women, and is most common when acquisition of HBV infection has been in childhood rather than adulthood. It is more common in cirrhotic patients, but may also occur in noncirrhotics. Viral integration within the chromosomes of hepatocytes may be an important pathogenic factor. Experimental evidence suggests that this induces changes in the host nucleus that predispose to carcinogenesis.

PRESENTATION

The clinical attack tends to be more severe for HBV than for other forms of hepatitis. In uncomplicated cases, the icteric phase usually lasts for 2–4 weeks, although rarely a prolonged cholestatic phase is observed. The clinical illness may be anicteric; such patients are more likely to develop chronic liver disease than those who develop jaundice. A minority of patients develop a serum sickness-like immune complex disease, which develops in the prodromal period. In this phase, transient rashes, arthritis, and, more rarely, arteritis or glomerulonephritis are observed.

Notes

INVESTIGATIONS

HBsAg usually appears in the serum about 6 weeks after infection and has disappeared by 12 weeks. Carrier state is defined by persistence of HBsAg for more than 6 months after the onset of symptoms. AntiHBs develops approximately 3 months after the onset and persists throughout life. Hepatitis B e antigen (HBeAg) is found in the serum of patients with ongoing viral replication and is a mark of infectivity and also of the development of chronic liver disease in patients who have the antigen present 10 weeks after the development of symptoms. Hepatitis B core antigen (HBcAg) is very rarely found in circulating blood, but antiHBc is detected frequently. High titres of IgM antiHBc represent an active viral infection, persistent lower titres usually indicate ongoing chronic disease. In the presence of antiHBs, low titres of IgG antiHBc represent past hepatitis B infection, whereas high titres without antiHBs indicate persistence of viral infection (*Table 37*). A direct evaluation of viral replication is the measurement of HBV DNA in the serum.

MANAGEMENT

There is no specific treatment for the acute phase of the disease. Not all patients with chronic hepatitis B infection are suitable for treatment. However, HBsAg-positive patients with circulating HBeAg should be considered for medical therapy, in order to reduce viral replication and hence infectivity. In addition, successful treatment may reduce the chance of progression to cirrhosis and liver failure.

Notes

Table 37 Guide to HBV serology

	AntiHBc IgM	AntiHBc IgG	HBeAg	HBsAg	AntiHBs
?Past infection		+ve			+ve, if virus cleared
?Acute hepatitis	+ve			+ve, may disappear within a few weeks	−ve
?Chronic hepatitis	−ve	+ve	+ve; if-ve, ?HBV mutant*, check HBV DNA by PCR	+ve	
?Carrier	−ve	+ve		+ve	
?Immune (postvaccination)					+ve (quantitative)

** A small proportion of patients with chronic active disease do not have detectable HBeAg because of genetic alteration of this protein antigen.*
PCR, polymerase chain reaction.

1.5

Standard treatment for hepatitis B consists of α-*interferon* in a dose of 5–10 million units three times weekly for 16 weeks given subcutaneously or intramuscularly. About 40% of patients will respond by loss of e antigen and conversion to e antibody, with a concomitant decrease in viral replication. Unfortunately no more than 10% of patients lose surface antigen and seroconvert to surface antibody indicating complete viral clearance. Factors such as sex, age, and race modify the response to α-interferon. Adverse effects, which are usually dose

Notes

related, include malaise, rigour, headaches, myalgia, fatigue, alopecia, depression, and bone marrow suppression. Fever, myalgia, and headache are usually worse with the first two or three injections of interferon, and tolerance usually develops. Elderly patients have a higher frequency of adverse effects. In a few cases the dose of α-interferon may need to be reduced in order to minimize adverse effects such as malaise and arthralgia which can be disabling. A minority of patients will develop antibodies to interferon but antiviral efficacy is not compromised.

Patients with severe hepatic decompensation such as ascites and encephalopathy should not be treated. Autoimmune diseases such as rheumatoid arthritis and thyroid disease may be exacerbated and they are also a contraindication to interferon therapy. In view of the relatively low response rate to interferon, other therapies, such as nucleoside analogues, are currently being assessed alone and in combination with interferon. Pretreatment with prednisolone to increase viral replication and hepatocyte damage has been used to increase the response rates to interferon, although not widely used as trials have been inconclusive.

Liver transplantation should be considered in patients with fulminant failure and in those with end-stage disease. Patients with end-stage liver disease and ongoing viral replication have a high risk of rapidly progressive liver injury from hepatitis B after transplantation. This risk can be reduced substantially by the prolonged use of high-dose hepatitis B immunoglobulin and possibly by the use of antivirals, such as lamivudine and famciclovir.

Notes

Prophylaxis

AntiHBs is the antibody responsible for immunity to HBV infection. Hepatitis B immunoglobulin (HBIG) is hyperimmune globulin with a high antibody titre of antiHBs antibody. It provides passive immunization. HBIG is used with a HBV vaccine for postexposure prophylaxis. To be effective HBIG (0.05 $ml\,kg^{-1}$ intramuscularly) is given within hours of potential infection, such as with a needlestick injury or sexual contacts of acute HBV. Hepatitis vaccine should be given within 7 days of exposure. This may not inhibit viral replication completely but may prevent severe illness or development of the carrier state. It is also essential that all babies of hepatitis B-positive mothers are given both passive (HBIG 100 units intramuscularly within 48 hours of birth) and active immunization following birth.

There are a number of commercially available *HBV vaccines*. These provide active immunity for more than 10 years. These vaccines are prepared from the non-infectious outer coat of the virus (HBsAg). Both the plasma-derived vaccine prepared from the plasma of HBV carriers and the recombinant vaccine are safe and both are highly effective (approximately 85% response rate over the age of 40 years, greater in those under 40) in preventing hepatitis B in high-risk patients. Response rates are lower in immunocompromised individuals. Indications for immunization are outlined in *Table 38* and dosage recommendations in *Table 39*.

Notes

Table 38 Indications for immunization against hepatitis B

Neonates of infected mothers (active and passive)
Accidental exposure (active and passive)
All healthcare personnel in frequent contact with blood or needles
Clients and staff of institutions for the intellectually disabled
Children in high-risk populations
Illicit intravenous drug use
Sex industry workers
Sexually active homosexual or bisexual men
Patients with chronic renal failure who are likely to need or require haemodialysis
Haemophiliacs
International travellers

Table 39 Hepatitis B vaccine dosage recommendations

	Engerix B	**Heptavax B (Recombivax HB)**
Adult dose	$\geqslant$ 19 years: 20 μg	$\geqslant$ 20 years: 10 μg
Adolescent dose	< 19 years: 10 μg	11–19 years: 5 μg
Pediatric dose		< 10 years: 2.5 μg (5 μg for neonates of HBsAg-positive mothers)
Schedule (intramuscular: deltoid or anterolateral aspect of thigh (infants))	0, 1 , and 6 months 0, 1, 2, and 12 months	0, 1 , and 6 months

Screening for hepatocellular carcinoma

Screening for hepatocellular carcinoma is appropriate for people at high risk. These include those aged over 40

Notes

years, of Asian or African background, with cirrhosis or a family history of hepatocellular carcinoma. Hepatic ultrasonography and estimation of serum α-fetoprotein levels at 3–6-monthly intervals are recommended.

1.5.10

Hepatitis D Virus (Delta Virus, HDV)

Delta agent is a small RNA strand coated with hepatitis B surface antigen (HBsAg), without which it is unable to replicate on its own and thus resembles the satellite viruses of plants, which cannot replicate without some other specific viral help. The hepatitis B and delta infection may be acquired simultaneously (coinfection) or the delta agent may infect a chronic HBsAg carrier (superinfection). Delta infection is worldwide; it is rare in the Far East and is particularly prevalent in illicit intravenous drug users, but it has been found in all the groups at high risk for hepatitis B.

PRESENTATION

The clinical picture of a coinfection is indistinguishable from that of hepatitis B, except that a biphasic rise in liver enzymes may be seen. The attack is usually self-limited as the delta agent cannot survive without persistent HBV surface antigenemia. The presence of delta predisposes to a fulminant course and one third of fulminant hepatitis B cases are related to coincidental delta infection. In the superinfection the attack is often severe and, again, may be fulminant or in some

Notes

asymptomatic, only shown by a rise in serum enzyme levels. Delta infection should always be excluded in any hepatitis B carrier who has a relapse of hepatitis. Although delta infection reduces hepatitis B viral replication, the presence of HDV usually worsens the course of chronic liver disease and may accelerate the progression to cirrhosis. Hepatocellular carcinoma is probably less common in HBsAg carriers with delta. It is unclear whether this represents inhibition by delta virus, or whether the patients die from worsening liver disease before the cancer can develop.

INVESTIGATIONS

Serum delta antigenemia is only present during the early stage of primary infection, before the development of antibody to HDV (antiHDV). Delta antigen (HDAg) can be demonstrated in hepatocytes during acute or chronic disease by immunohistologic techniques. Screening for HDV relies on indirect antibody (IgM/IgG antiHD) testing. These antibodies are not protective and coexist with chronic disease.

MANAGEMENT

Immunosuppressive therapy is not helpful in delta virus infection. Clinical trials with interferon have shown transient inhibition of delta replication with a fall in serum transaminase concentration, but these changes reverse rapidly on stopping treatment. Hepatic transplantation has given poor results as rapid recurrence of both hepatitis B and delta virus occurs in the transplanted liver.

Notes

Prophylaxis

In patients who have not been infected with hepatitis B, full protection from delta virus infection is provided by hepatitis B vaccination (see *1.5.9 Hepatitis B (HBV Hepatitis)*). There is no available vaccine against delta virus infection for hepatitis B carriers.

1.5.11

Hepatitis C (HCV Hepatitis)

Serologic tests for hepatitis A and B viruses became available in 1974. Other viral agent(s) were clearly responsible for many cases of hepatitis, particularly those following blood transfusion. NonA nonB (NANB) hepatitis was the classification, but in 1989 the nucleic acid of hepatitis C virus was isolated.

EPIDEMIOLOGY AND PATHOGENESIS

HCV is a single-stranded RNA virus of about 10 000 base pairs in length. The prevalence in developed countries is between 1 and 8 per 1000 population. There is a high prevalence in haemophiliacs, thalassaemics, intravenous drug abusers, and haemodialysed patients infected by transfusion of blood or blood products. Nonparenteral transmission is well recognized but sexual and maternal–infant transmission is rare. The carriage rate in undeveloped countries can be as high as 20%.

There is considerable nucleotide variation of the HCV genome, which has resulted in the classification of HCV

Notes

into six main genotypes (nucleotide variation greater than 30% over the complete genome), with further division into closely related subtypes (differing by more than 20% in the sequence). Geographic differences in the distribution of viral genotypes probably reflect the epidemiologic history of the virus. Genotypes 1, 2, and 3 account for the majority of HCV infections in western Europe, North America, and Australia. Subtypes also vary in their geographic distribution: subtype 1a is common in western Europe and North America, whereas type 1b is more likely to occur in eastern and southern Europe and in Asia.

The incubation period is 8 weeks with a range of 2–26 weeks. Despite the benign acute course, approximately 80% of patients progress to chronic hepatitis and subsequently to cirrhosis and hepatocellular carcinoma (HCC) (see *Figure 7*). In patients who develop cirrhosis the average duration of chronic hepatitis has been about 12–15 years. Factors that may interact with HCV in leading to HCC include chronic liver disease, hepatitis B virus, alcohol, and iron overload. The cumulative 10-year rate of development of HCC in patients with HCV cirrhosis is about 60%. This increases to about 80% if both heavy alcohol intake and HCV cirrhosis are present, compared with about 20% for cirrhosis and heavy alcohol intake alone.

PRESENTATION

Clinical features of acute HCV infection overlap with those of HAV and HBV infections (see *1.5.8* and *1.5.9*). Symptoms, if present, are usually mild and anicteric

Notes

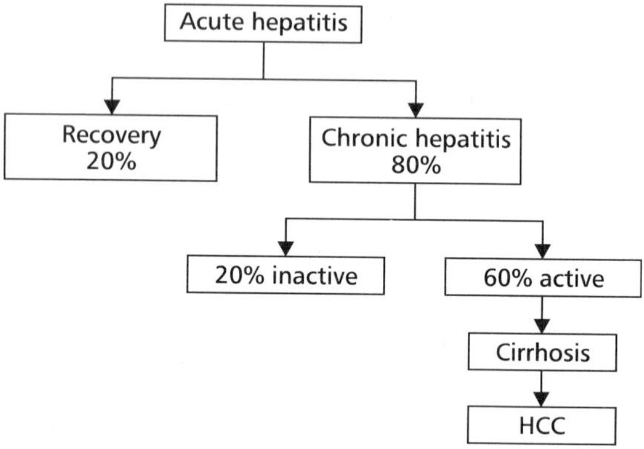

Figure 7 Outcome of acute hepatitis C infection.

hepatitis is common, although transaminase (aminotransferase) levels can fluctuate. Acute HCV disease is less severe than HAV or HBV. Most infected individuals fail to clear the virus and will have changes of chronic hepatitis on liver biopsy by 6 months of infection. Serum levels of transaminases may be normal or mildly abnormal. In the longer term, symptoms (especially tiredness) and transaminase levels may fluctuate widely. Many patients are not recognized until they present with signs of chronic liver disease associated with HCV cirrhosis.

Hepatitis C has also been associated with autoimmune liver disease, thyroiditis, essential mixed cryoglobulinemia, membranoproliferative glomerulonephritis, and porphyria cutanea tarda.

Notes

INVESTIGATIONS

Fluctuating increases in the levels of transaminases are characteristic, but histologic features of macrovesicular fatty liver, bile duct damage, and lymphocytic infiltration are also common. There are many enzyme-linked immunosorbent assays (ELISAs) for antibodies to nonstructural antigens of HCV. Antibodies can also be confirmed by a recombinant immunoblot assay (RIBA). It may be as much as 6 months before antibodies appear in the serum. The polymerase chain reaction (PCR) for HCV RNA is essential for confirming HCV infection.

MANAGEMENT

Acute hepatitis C

The management of acute sporadic or transfusion-related hepatitis C consists of conventional supportive management of acute liver disease and specific antiviral therapy in selected cases. Specific antiviral therapy consists of treatment with *α-interferon* in a dose of 3–6 million units three times a week subcutaneously for 12 weeks (see *2.3.1 Interferon*). Recent trials show a response rate of 60–80% with lowering of transaminase levels and clearance of the HCV. Complete clearance of the virus appears to occur in about 20% of patients. Further studies are needed to identify patients who would otherwise progress to chronic liver disease and are thus candidates for early interferon therapy.

Notes

1.5

Chronic hepatitis C

An algorithm for the use of interferon in patients with chronic HCV is presented in *Figure 8*. It remains controversial which patients should be offered such therapy. Other forms of chronic viral hepatitis and autoimmune hepatitis should be excluded prior to interferon treatment. Interferon may exacerbate the clinical manifestations of all autoimmune diseases. Liver biopsy should be performed because there is a poor correlation between enzyme levels and histologic liver damage.

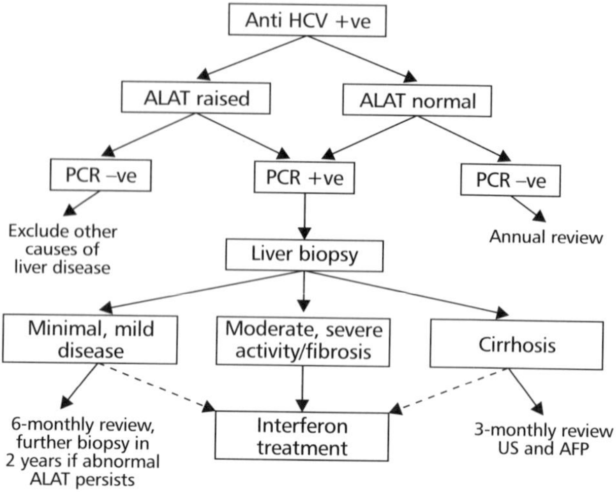

Figure 8 Hepatitis C algorithm. ALAT, alanine aminotransferase; PCR, polymerase chain reaction; US, ultrasonography; AFP, α-fetoprotein. Adapted from Booth *et al. Gut* 1995; **37**: 451 (with permission).

Notes

Therapeutic trials of *α-interferon* show that 50% of patients will have a normal serum aminotransferase level after treatment courses with 3 million units three times a week by intramuscular or subcutaneous injection for 6 months. After stopping treatment, however, half will relapse. Some 20% have a prolonged response to therapy and do not again develop raised levels of aminotransferases and remain negative for HCV RNA. Of more clinical importance, however, is emerging evidence that the rate of development of cirrhosis may be reduced by interferon therapy. Current clinical trials are examining longer durations of treatment with α-interferon (>12 months) and the combination of α-interferon with antivirals such as ribraviron. There is also some evidence that higher doses of α-interferon may be more effective.

The genotype of the hepatitis C virus appears to be an important predictor of response. The presence of genotype 1b is associated with a poor response. This may partly reflect the duration of infectivity and viral load. Patients who are already cirrhotic have a poor biochemical/RNA response and are not currently offered treatment. There is preliminary evidence, however, that interferon treatment in cirrhotics may reduce the occurrence of HCC.

Patients with a normal serum ALAT concentration and who are negative for HCV RNA 1 year after stopping therapy can be considered to have cleared HCV.

Liver transplantation

Cirrhosis due to hepatitis C is a common indication for liver transplantation. However, recurrence of hepatitis

Notes

C virus is common and 90% of all patients transplanted will become HCV RNA positive once more within 2 weeks of the transplant, but is associated with mild disease. Interferon may increase rejection and other antiviral agents are on trial.

Screening for hepatocellular carcinoma

Screening for HCC is appropriate for people with cirrhosis secondary to hepatitis C. Hepatic ultrasonography and estimation of serum α-fetoprotein levels at 3–6-monthly intervals are recommended.

1.5.12

Hepatitis E (HEV Hepatitis)

The etiological agent of epidemic nonA nonB hepatitis is a virus-like particle (HEV) with biophysical and biochemical characteristics of calciviruses.

PRESENTATION

The clinical course closely resembles that of hepatitis A. It affects mainly young adults, causing a short-lived hepatitis. Huge epidemics of HEV hepatitis have been reported from India, Pakistan, Russia, and South-East Asia. It does not progress to chronic liver disease, but there is a high mortality rate in women in the last trimester of pregnancy (20%).

Notes

INVESTIGATIONS

Serologic tests for seroconversion to HEV are available. HEV RNA can be detected in blood and stool by the polymerase chain reaction.

MANAGEMENT

There is no known treatment, but as the virus is spread by the faecal–oral route, prevention depends on the provision of a clean water supply and adequate sanitation.

1.5.13

Pyogenic Liver Abscess

In the developed world liver abscesses are uncommon, but they are seen frequently in developing countries, causing acute and chronic illness.

EPIDEMIOLOGY AND PATHOGENESIS

Ascending infection with portal pyemia from intra-abdominal sepsis is the most common cause. This can arise from an appendiceal or diverticular abscess, although in many cases the etiology is not clear. In elderly patients biliary sepsis causing ascending cholangitis is a common cause. The commonest organisms are enteric in origin (e.g. *Escherichia coli*, *Streptococcus faecalis* and *Proteus vulgaris*. *Streptococcus milleri* and anaerobic organisms such as *Bacteroides* are now more frequently seen and, in view of the pathogenesis, it is not surprising that the infections

Notes

are often mixed. In developed countries abscesses due to *S. milleri* are associated with colonic neoplasia.

PRESENTATION

Patients can present an insidious chronic course with malaise and low-grade fever lasting for several weeks or months before the diagnosis is established. Alternatively they present acutely with fever, rigours, anorexia, weight loss, and right upper quadrant pain which may radiate to the back. On examination there may be no abnormal findings, but some patients are febrile and jaundiced, with an enlarged tender liver.

INVESTIGATIONS

Liver function test results can be completely normal, but the most common abnormality is a raised serum alkaline phosphatase level. In less than a quarter of patients, other changes in serum liver biochemistry are seen. The white cell count is usually raised showing a polymorph leucocytosis with a high C-reactive protein level and ESR. Blood cultures are diagnostic in only one third of cases. A high clinical index of suspicion is required.

The mainstay of diagnosis is imaging by ultrasonography and computed tomography, allowing diagnostic and therapeutic aspiration at the same time.

MANAGEMENT

Therapeutic aspiration should be attempted if the abscess is greater than 2 cm and broad-spectrum antibiotics

Notes

should be administered intravenously until the causative organism has been isolated. Rarely, open surgical drainage will be required in patients in whom radiologic aspiration has proved to be unsuccessful. In addition, the underlying causes should be sought and treated. The prognosis is dependent on the cause of the liver abscess and the underlying state of the patient. In general, scattered multiple abscesses are associated with a higher mortality rate than single lesions.

1.5.14

Amoebic Abscess

EPIDEMIOLOGY AND PATHOGENESIS

This is common in developing countries and must be considered in developed countries in patients traveling from endemic areas. The infection with *Entamoeba histolytica* ascends from colonic infection to the liver via the portal venous system. This causes the formation of multiple microabscesses which coalesce to form a single abscess or multiple large abscesses.

PRESENTATION

The onset of symptoms is usually insidious with fever, anorexia, weight loss, and malaise. Characteristically, there is no previous history of amoebic dysentery. On examination there is evidence of hepatomegaly with tenderness in the right upper quadrant. A firm thump over the lower chest often provokes pain. Jaundice is rare.

Notes

INVESTIGATIONS

The investigations are as for pyogenic liver abscess (see *1.5.13*), except that in patients who are at risk serologic tests for amoeba should be sent (amoebic fluorescent antibody test). While a positive result does not indicate clinical disease, and antibodies may remain for months after a clinical cure, a negative test is good evidence against ongoing amoebic infection. Aspiration is usually diagnostic producing fluid looking like "anchovy sauce".

MANAGEMENT

The treatment is diagnostic aspiration together with antibiotic therapy. In suspected amoebic abscess, metronidazole should be used in a dose of 800 mg three times daily for 10 days (see also *1.4.5.1.2 Entamoeba histolytica*). In view of the risk of mixed infection, broad-spectrum antibiotics are usually added to the metronidazole. Rarely, the cysts may rupture to the pulmonary space or peritoneum.

1.5.15

Hydatid Disease

EPIDEMIOLOGY AND PATHOGENESIS

Hydatid cysts can occur worldwide, through ingestion of embryos of the dog tapeworm (*Echinococcus granulosus* or *Echinococcus multilocularis*). The disease is seen particularly

Notes

in sheep and cattle farming communities. Inside the human gut the embryos hatch, penetrate the intestinal wall, and enter the portal system and then the liver. They may be further disseminated through the lungs into any organ of the body, causing problems of a space-occupying lesion. The liver is the commonest site for cyst formation (60% of infected patients), which usually develop in the right lobe. The cyst consists of an outside layer derived from the host, an intermediate layer, and an inner germinal centre which buds off brood capsules to form daughter cysts.

PRESENTATION

Patients may frequently be asymptomatic but some present with the space-occupying lesion in the right hypochondrium. Dead cysts become calcified, so may be found on routine radiography. Complications may occur from space-occupying lesions in the brain and, rarely, cysts may rupture into the pulmonary tree.

INVESTIGATIONS

Blood films may show an eosinophilia, and the hydatid complement fixation test is usually positive. Scanning by ultrasonography and computed tomography usually demonstrates a multilayered cyst suggesting the diagnosis. As a general rule, needle aspiration should not be performed because of the risk of dissemination of the hydatid disease and anaphylactic shock. Fine-needle aspiration performed under chemotherapeutic cover is not recommended outside tertiary referral centres.

Notes

MANAGEMENT

Treatment consists of surgical removal of the cyst, usually after injecting the cyst with formalin to sterilize it before handling. Medical treatment with albendazole is used in some cases, although results are variable.

1.5.16

Alcoholic Liver Disease

EPIDEMIOLOGY AND PATHOGENESIS

Some 10–15% of people who abuse alcohol (alcoholics) develop liver disease. There is a genetic predisposition and females are more liable than males to develop liver disease. Alcohol abuse can be defined as an established pattern of regular alcohol consumption in excess of 60 g daily for men and of 40 g daily for women. Of note, however, is that liver injury can occur with regular intake of lesser amounts of alcohol: the relative risk of cirrhosis is six times greater at 40–60 g daily than at 0–20 g daily, and 14 times greater at 60–80 g daily; in women the risk increases with alcohol intake over 20 g daily. Although unproven, hepatitis B or C infection and α_1-antitrypsin deficiency may also act as cofactors in the development of alcohol-related liver disease.

Acetaldehyde, the product of hepatic ethanol oxidation, is thought to be responsible for many of the toxic effects of alcohol. Damage includes changes in the intracellular redox potential, protein retention in the hepatocyte, increased liver fat, the induction of a

Notes

hypermetabolic state, and effects on the immune system. Alcohol produces a wide spectrum of morphologic liver damage, the main subtypes being fatty liver, alcoholic hepatitis, and cirrhosis (*Figure 9*).

Fatty liver (steatosis)

Alcohol causes macrovesicular fat which can be throughout the hepatic lobule. This is the earliest manifestation of alcohol-related liver injury and the most frequently seen pattern of injury. Commonly, small droplet or microvesicular fat is also seen. These changes are nonspecific and are seen in diabetes mellitus, obesity, starvation, and inflammatory bowel disease (see *1.5.17 Nonalcoholic Fatty Liver*). This lesion is not usually precirrhotic and reverses on stopping alcohol. Fatty liver may be associated with perivenular fibrosis, which may indicate individuals at higher risk of progression to cirrhosis if drinking continues.

Alcoholic hepatitis

Alcoholic hepatitis is characterized by hepatocyte degeneration and necrosis with lobular infiltration with neutrophils and the presence of Mallory's hyaline. Both macrovesicular and microvesicular steatosis are also frequently present. Perivenular and pericellular ("chicken-wire") fibrosis seen in association with alcoholic

Alcohol-related fatty liver → Alcoholic hepatitis (subclinical or clinical) → Cirrhosis

Figure 9 The progression of alcohol-related liver injury.

Notes

hepatitis is highly characteristic of alcohol-related liver injury and indicates that progression to cirrhosis is likely, particularly if alcohol consumption continues.

Alcoholic cirrhosis

Ongoing hepatitis and fibrosis will eventually disrupt the normal acinar architecture of the liver with the development of small regenerative nodules (micronodular cirrhosis). The cirrhotic process may be macronodular especially if the patient becomes abstinent. A mixed pattern of macronodular and micronodular cirrhosis is also frequently found. Cirrhosis is not a reversible process, although abstinence can improve survival. Subsequent to the development of a macroregenerative cirrhosis, however, is an increased risk of hepatocellular carcinoma.

Prognosis depends on abstinence from alcohol. Decompensated cirrhotics have a 5-year survival rate of 50%. Alcoholic hepatitis often gets worse during the first few weeks in hospital despite abstinence, and complete resolution may take up to 6 months, with a mortality rate of up to 50%.

PRESENTATION

Patients with alcoholic liver disease most commonly are either asymptomatic at presentation, their finding of liver disease being coincidental, or they present with non-specific symptoms such as abdominal pain, vomiting, anorexia, diarrhoea, weight loss, lethargy, and fatigue. Presentation with features of decompensated liver dis-

Notes

ease such as jaundice, ascites, or gastrointestinal bleeding is less common.

Patients with fatty liver are usually asymptomatic. An enlarged, smooth, firm liver is often palpable and there may be mild increases in the level of aminotransferases (ALAT, ASAT). Occasionally patients with fatty liver present with hepatomegaly and symptoms of intrahepatic cholestasis. There may be a marked transient increase of the ALAT concentration, with a more prolonged increase in the level of alkaline phosphatase and bilirubin. This pattern differs from that of alcoholic hepatitis and may mimic extrahepatic biliary obstruction. Liver biopsy usually shows large amounts of both microvesicular and macrovesicular fat together with cholestasis; there is little or no fibrosis or inflammation.

The clinical picture is variable in patients with alcoholic hepatitis. In mild to moderate cases fatigue, anorexia, and weight loss with a large tender liver are characteristic. Life-threatening decompensation and failure occurs in severe disease. The patient is ill, jaundiced, and often has ascites. Right upper quadrant abdominal pain is associated with a high fever. Signs of chronic liver disease are usually present; particularly impressive are spider nevi and palmar erythema.

Some patients presenting with established cirrhosis may give no preceding history of acute alcoholic hepatitis and have few symptoms. Signs of chronic liver disease, including splenomegaly, alert the physician to the diagnosis following presentation with complications of severe liver disease.

The possibility of alcoholic liver disease may arise in patients referred because of a drinking problem or

Notes

because of the development of withdrawal symptoms when they are admitted to hospital for a nonliver illness. They could also present with pancreatitis or peripheral neuropathy. Pancreatitis may be associated with cholestasis because of compression of the common bile duct by an inflamed pancreas (see *1.6.1 Acute Pancreatitis* or *1.6.2 Chronic Pancreatitis*).

Withdrawal symptoms are most likely to occur with complete or partial abstinence of alcohol after prolonged and regular heavy intake. Manifestations include tremour, hallucinations, withdrawal seizures, and delerium tremens. Increasing tremour appears 12–24 hours after the last drink and may be associated with restlessness, agitation, and insomnia. It takes hours to days to subside. Visual and auditory hallucinations can occur within a few days of alcohol withdrawal. Generalized epileptic seizures, occasionally status epilepticus, are uncommon but may occur 12–48 hours after alcohol withdrawal. Delerium tremens is a withdrawal syndrome that occurs in 5 % or less of individuals withdrawing from alcohol. It is characterized by coarse tremour, restlessness, profound confusion, delusions, and hallucinations. Autonomic manifestations include sweating, tachycardia, skin flushing or pallor, and fever.

INVESTIGATIONS

A drinking history is important in order to establish whether an individual has regularly consumed an amount of alcohol that can potentially cause harm. An inventory of major life events that may trigger or be associated with alcoholism is also important. Symptoms

Notes

of physical dependency should be sought. Corroboration from people who know the individual in question should be sought.

A raised breath or blood ethanol concentration may draw attention to the possibility of alcohol abuse, but is of limited diagnostic value in the actual assessment of liver disease.

Biochemical aberrations, although not specific, frequently occur with alcohol abuse. The serum γ-glutamyl transpeptidase (γGT) is a sensitive test for alcohol abuse (the enzyme is induced by regular alcohol intake) but raised levels do not necessarily indicate liver damage. Serum transaminase levels are usually either normal or only mildly increased, even when marked hepatic inflammation is present. The aspartate to alanine aminotransferase ratio (ASAT:ALAT) is often greater than 2. Alkaline phosphatase concentration may be increased (more than three times normal), particularly in those with cholestatic syndromes.

Depressed hepatic synthetic function is indicated by a low serum albumin concentration and prolonged prothrombin time (international normalized ratio (INR)). These, together with serum bilirubin levels, indicate the severity of the damage and are often used in scoring the severity of liver disease (see *Table 40*). Such a score is a useful prognostic indicator in alcoholic and nonalcoholic cirrhosis.

A raised serum immunoglobulin (Ig) A level often occurs with alcohol abuse, especially when cirrhosis is present. It may remain increased for many months following abstinence. In alcoholic hepatitis a neutrophil leucocytosis, seen in approximately one third of patients,

Notes

Table 40 Child–Pugh grading of severity of liver disease

Clinical or biochemical measurement	Points scored for increasing abnormality		
	1	2	3
Encephalopathy (see Table 28, page 227)	None	Grades 1 and 2	Grades 3, 4, or 5
Ascites	Absent	Slight	Moderate
Bilirubin (mg per 100 ml)	1–2	2–3	> 3
Albumin ($g\,l^{-1}$)	> 35	28–35	< 28
Prothrombin (seconds prolonged)	1–4	4–6	> 6
For primary biliary cirrhosis, bilirubin (mg per 100 ml)	1–4	4–10	> 10

Grade A, score 5–7; grade B, score 8–10; grade C, score 11–15.

1.5

is marker of disease severity. The mean corpuscular volume (MCV) is commonly raised due either to alcohol *per se* or secondary to chronic liver disease and folate deficiency.

There is no one laboratory test that can act as a "gold standard" for the detection of alcohol abuse. However, the combination of several tests (such as γGT, ASAT (or ASAT:ALAT ratio) and MCV) can have a high sensitivity and specificity.

Fatty liver is detectable by ultrasonography, computed tomography or magnetic resonance imaging when macrovesicular steatosis is present in more than 50% of hepatocytes. Fibrosis, however, is less reliably detected.

Notes

A liver biopsy should be done in all individuals who are actively abusing alcohol and who have hepatomegaly and/or abnormal liver function test results. The main reason for a biopsy is to identify accurately the cause of the underlying liver disease. In about 30% of patients there will either be a nonalcoholic cause for the liver disease or the injury will be due to a combination of alcohol and a nonalcoholic cause. These nonalcoholic causes, such as genetic haemochromatosis, may require specific treatment; this could prevent or slow the progression of liver injury. Other reasons for liver biopsy include assessment of the stage and severity of liver disease and evaluation for/of therapy.

MANAGEMENT

There are a number of different manifestations of alcohol abuse which require different management strategies. Immediate and continued abstinence from alcohol is the most important therapeutic measure in any of these strategies.

Alcohol withdrawal

Moderate to severe alcohol withdrawal symptoms should be treated with chlormethiazole or benzodiazepines, such as chlordiazepoxide. Chlormethiazole can be given orally or, if delerium tremens or seizures are present, intravenously. Oral dosage is two to four capsules on admission and a further two capsules hourly until adequately sedated (maximum of eight capsules in the first 2 hours). The chlormethiazole is subsequently titrated to the patient's response, up to a maximum of 16

Notes

capsules per day. The dose should be gradually decreased over about 10 days. Intravenous chlormethiazole is infused at an initial rate of 12–20 mg per min until shallow sleep, reducing to 4–6 mg per min for maintenance, to achieve the lowest possible rate to maintain shallow sleep and good spontaneous breathing. The patient can be converted subsequently to oral chlormethiazole. Following discharge from hospital skilled psychiatric help may be required to maintain remission from alcohol abuse.

Alcoholic hepatitis

In patients with alcoholic hepatitis a period of hospitalization is usually required. Complications of decompensated liver disease such as bleeding, infection, ascites, or encephalopathy may require specific treatment (see *1.5.1–1.5.4*). Nutritional deficiencies should be corrected. Ongoing maintenance of a good nutritional intake is important and may require nasogastric, or even intravenous, nutrition.

Several experimental therapies have been evaluated aimed at stabilizing patients during the acute phase of alcoholic hepatitis. These therapies include corticosteroids, to reduce immunologic injury; propylthiouracil, given to decrease the hypermetabolic state and reduce perivenular (zone 3) hypoxia; insulin and glucagon, to stimulate hepatic regeneration; and anabolic steroids, to promote an anabolic state. With the exception of corticosteroids, none has been shown to reduce mortality. Recent studies have suggested that corticosteroid therapy (prednisolone 40 mg per day for 1 month) can reduce

Notes

short-term mortality in patients with biopsy-proven severe alcoholic hepatitis manifested by spontaneous hepatic encephalopathy or a markedly prolonged prothrombin time with a greatly increased bilirubin concentration[1], and neutrophilia with a hepatic polymorphonuclear leucocyte infiltrate. The 1-year survival rate can be improved from about 40% to about 70% in such patients. It is usually not appropriate to consider patients for liver transplantation during the acute phase of their illness. However, after 6–12 months of abstinence the patient's condition may indicate that transplantation is appropriate.

Cirrhosis

Management of the complications of decompensated liver disease, with or without cirrhosis, is covered elsewhere (see *1.5.1–1.5.4*). In patients who are clinically stable, hepatocellular carcinoma is a significant long-term risk; hepatic ultrasonography and estimation of serum α-foetoprotein levels at 3–6-monthly intervals may be appropriate.

Patients with alcohol-related cirrhosis form one of the largest groups evaluated for liver transplantation. The majority of patients have Child–Pugh grade B or C disease, and medical supportive measures have failed. An arbitrary 6-month abstinence period has been required by some centers. There can be a remarkable improvement in patients over such a period, especially

[1] High risk if the discriminant function: 4.6 (prothrombin time − control time (seconds) + serum bilirubin ($\mu mol\ l^{-1}$)/17 is greater than 32.

Notes

in those with alcoholic hepatitis. This may delay the need for transplantation. Some patients, however, will be too sick to be likely to survive such a trial period and or decision will need to be made whether to transplant early or not. Recidivism following transplant is between 9 and 33%.

1.5.17

Nonalcoholic Fatty Liver

There is a group of entities in which the histologic features of the liver may resemble, but are not due to, those of alcohol. There are three main histologic patterns that resemble phases of alcoholic liver disease: nonalcoholic steatosis (fatty liver); nonalcoholic steatohepatitis (NASH) in which the fat is associated with inflammation, with or without Mallory bodies; and nonalcoholic steatocirrhosis.

EPIDEMIOLOGY AND PATHOGENESIS

The main clinical associations of nonalcoholic fatty liver are shown in *Table 41*. Steatosis, which is mainly macrovesicular, is the most common lesion. In some this may progress to steatohepatitis and rarely to cirrhosis. The likelihood of such progression is greater in obese patients if diabetes is present, and greater still if both these conditions are associated with a surgical jejunoileal bypass. Up to 50% of patients undergoing intestinal bypass may have a deterioration of hepatic function with liver histopathology resembling alcoholic hepatitis or alcoholic cirrhosis.

Notes

Table 41 Major clinical associations of nonalcoholic fatty liver

Cause	Findings
"Acquired" metabolic	Obesity Diabetes mellitus (type II) Intestinal bypass, especially jejunoileal bypass Protein calorie malnutrition Total parenteral nutrition Inflammatory bowel disease
Drugs and toxins	Amiodarone Methotrexate Perhexiline maleate 4,4′-Diethylaminoethoxyhexestrol Wilson's disease Indian childhood cirrhosis
Miscellaneous	Chronic hepatitis C

PRESENTATION

Seventy-five per cent or more patients are female and more than 70% of patients are obese. Most patients are only about 30–40% overweight. Diabetes mellitus is present in more than 30% of patients. The majority of cases are asymptomatic, and most come to medical attention because of hepatomegaly and/or minor hepatic enzyme abnormality.

INVESTIGATIONS

Levels of liver enzymes are usually only mildly raised with the serum aspartate and alanine aminotransferases (ASAT and ALAT) usually less than five times normal

Notes

and the alkaline phosphatase level two times the normal value, or less. Serum albumin levels and prothrombin time are almost always normal. Hepatic steatosis (fatty liver) has a characteristic appearance on ultrasonography (bright echogenic pattern), computed tomography or magnetic resonance imaging. The definitive diagnosis and evaluation require liver biopsy.

MANAGEMENT

Simple fatty liver is a benign condition which usually resolves if the underlying clinical cause is treated. Modest weight reduction should be achieved gradually. Rapid weight reduction may be associated with a deterioration in hepatic function. Patients with a jejuno-ileal bypass have been treated by reversal of the bypass or with metronidazole or other antibiotics to prevent intestinal bacterial overgrowth (see *1.4.15*)

1.5.18

Primary Biliary Cirrhosis

Primary biliary cirrhosis (PBC) is a chronic progressive disorder that is characterized by progressive destruction of the small intralobular bile ducts leading to cholestasis, portal inflammation, and scarring, and eventually to cirrhosis and liver failure.

EPIDEMIOLOGY AND PATHOGENESIS

The etiology is unknown, but immunologic mechanisms play a major role. The disease is characterized by the

Notes

presence of antibodies to mitochondria (AMA) and the antigens have been further identified as enzymes of the pyruvate dehydrogenase complex of the inner mitochondrial membrane. The importance of the antimitochondrial antibodies in the pathogenesis is unclear because there is no correlation between the AMA titre and the severity or rate of progression of PBC. Bile duct destruction is mediated through sensitized T lymphocytes. This may be triggered by antigenic expression on the basolateral membrane of biliary epithelial cells.

There are some patients with the clinicopathologic features of PBC who are negative for AMA, but either positive or negative for antinuclear antibody (ANA). In some of these the AMA titre goes from negative to positive, or from positive to negative, over the course of the disease. The term "autoimmune cholangitis" (AMA^+ or AMA^-) has been thus proposed as an alternative name for the group as a whole, including those with all the features of PBC.

PRESENTATION

PBC predominantly affects middle-aged women with a female to male ratio of 9:1. The early symptoms are of malaise, right upper quadrant discomfort, and pruritus which may progress to jaundice, usually over many years. In the later stages there are features of chronic liver disease with hepatosplenomegaly, pigmentation xanthalasmata, and cutaneous xanthomas. There is a close relationship with other organ-specific autoimmune disorders, particularly keratoconjunctivitis sicca, scleroderma, rheumatoid arthritis, autoimmune thyroiditis, renal tubular acidosis,

Notes

and glomerulonephritis. Breast cancer and urinary infection are also more common in these patients.

INVESTIGATIONS

Increased serum levels of IgM are found in most patients and most have high titres of many autoantibodies, such as ANAs, AMAs, and antithyroid antibodies. AMAs are present in the serum of over 95% of patients. Serum biochemistry indicates cholestasis with a predominantly high alkaline phosphatase level. Liver histology reveals, in the early stages, a portal infiltrate of lymphocytes and plasma cells with granulomata closely associated with the intrahepatic bile ducts. As the disease progresses bile ducts are lost, exacerbating cholestasis and eventually causing fibrosis and cirrhosis.

MANAGEMENT

Management should control symptoms but there is also specific treatment for PBC. The pruritus is usually treated with cholestyramine 2 g (half a sachet) before and after breakfast initially, increasing to up to four sachets daily until the pruritus is controlled. Alternative bile salt-binding agents can be used, such as colestipol if cholestyramine is too unpalatable. Alternative medical therapies for pruritus include rifampicin and naltrexone 50 mg b.i.d. Malabsorption of fat-soluble vitamins A, D and K occurs and intramuscular supplements are required. Oral calcium supplements can be given; the role of hormone replacement therapy and etidronate in the treatment of osteoporosis remain to be determined.

Notes

Specific therapy for primary biliary cirrhosis is *ursodeoxycholic acid* in a dose of 10–15 mg per kg weight. Ursodeoxycholic acid significantly prolongs the time before liver transplantation is needed or reduces the likelihood of death. The role of other agents such as colchicine and methotrexate remains to be determined by clinical trials, which are in progress. PBC has been shown to respond favourably to corticosteroids, but accelerated bone loss contraindicates this therapy. Liver transplantation remains the only treatment for patients with advanced chronic liver disease.

1.5.19

Autoimmune Hepatitis

Autoimmune hepatitis is characterized by hypergammaglobulinemia, autoantibodies in serum, and the presence on liver biopsy of, at least, periportal hepatitis (interface hepatitis or piecemeal necrosis). Chronicity is the usual feature, and may have an acute, even fulminant, presentation. Autoimmune hepatitis was formerly called lupoid hepatitis or autoimmune chronic active hepatitis.

EPIDEMIOLOGY AND PATHOGENESIS

The triggering factor for this immune-mediated liver disease is unknown. The disease is characterized by destruction of hepatocytes by activated T lymphocytes. There is a close association with other organ-specific autoimmune diseases such as autoimmune thyroiditis and Coombs-positive haemolytic anaemia. Approximately

Notes

60% of patients have the HLA haplotype A1 B8 DR3 and there is a separate association with DR4.

PRESENTATION

Autoimmune hepatitis occurs most frequently in women less than 40 years old, especially in the second decade. The onset is usually insidious with malaise, arthralgia, and jaundice, but about a quarter of patients present with acute hepatitis. Clinical examination may reveal signs of chronic liver disease as well as cutaneous striae, acne, and hirsutism. About 25% of patients have cirrhosis at presentation, indicating that the disease often has an indolent but aggressive subclinical phase.

INVESTIGATIONS

Serum biochemistry is characterized by an increase in the levels of autoantibodies, immunoglobulins (more than 1.5 times the normal value), and aminotransferases. In the absence of markers of active viral infections; denial of parenteral exposure to blood or blood products; absence of other etiologic factors such as excess alcohol, the diagnosis is reasonably established by high titres (at least 1:80) of antinuclear antibodies (ANAs), and smooth muscle antibodies (SMAs). A subgroup of young patients may have liver–kidney microsomal type 1 antibodies (antiLKM1). Liver histology shows interface hepatitis (piecemeal necrosis), fibrosis, and occasionally cirrhosis; there are no biliary lesions, granulomas, excess iron or copper, or other histologic features suggestive of a different etiology.

Notes

MANAGEMENT

Initial treatment is with oral *prednisolone* 30 mg daily for 2 weeks. The dose is reduced to a maintenance dose of 7.5–10 mg daily which is maintained for 2 years. A minority of patients can be weaned off immunosuppressive therapy completely, the majority will relapse and require further long-term immunosuppression. Patients in whom the dose of prednisolone cannot be reduced below 10 mg, or in whom profound steroidal side-effects develop, can be treated with *azathioprine* in a maximal dose of 2 mg per kg. In severely compromised patients who do not respond within 2 weeks of starting treatment, liver transplantation should be considered and the diagnosis reassessed. Other drugs under investigation include ursodeoxycholic acid, cyclosporin, and FK506.

1.5.20

Primary Sclerosing Cholangitis

Primary sclerosing cholangitis (PSC) is a chronic inflammatory disorder causing stricturing and fibrosis of intrahepatic and extrahepatic biliary bile ducts leading to fibrosis and biliary cirrhosis.

EPIDEMIOLOGY AND PATHOGENESIS

About 5–10% of patients with inflammatory bowel disease will develop PSC. Conversely, approximately 70% of patents with PSC have inflammatory bowel

Notes

disease. PSC occurs more often in ulcerative colitis than in Crohn's disease.

The etiology is unknown although immune factors are thought to be important. There is a close association with an HLA-B8 DR3 haplotype and it is probable that the bile duct loss is T-cell mediated.

PRESENTATION

The condition is most commonly seen in young male patients with a male : female predominance of 2 : 1. The majority of patients are asymptomatic at presentation and are found to have high alkaline phosphatase levels in the presence of ulcerative colitis. However, about 10–15% of patients present with recurrent fever, right upper quadrant pain, pruritus, malaise, and jaundice. Clinical examination may reveal evidence of chronic liver disease, although this is rarely present in the early stages of the condition.

INVESTIGATIONS

Biochemical tests usually indicate a cholestasis, although this typically may be fluctuant. Serum autoantibodies reveal a positive perinuclear antineutrophil cytoplasmic antibody (pANCA) in two thirds of patients as well as an increase in serum levels of IgM in jaundiced patients. Liver biopsy may show evidence of portal infiltration and concentric fibrosis around bile ducts in early cases, progressing in later stages to bile duct loss, fibrosis, and cirrhosis. The gold standard for diagnosis is endoscopic retrograde cholangiopancreatography (ERCP) which

Notes

reveals stricturing and dilatation, usually of both the intrahepatic and extrahepatic biliary trees. The strict definition requires that gallstones are not found.

MANAGEMENT

Cholestasis is treated in the same way as for primary biliary cirrhosis (see *1.5.18*). There is no medical therapy shown to alter the natural history of PSC, although *ursodeoxycholic acid* (10–15 mg per kg body weight orally per day in divided doses) is clearly associated with biochemical improvement. About 10–20% of patients will develop cholangiocarcinoma, for which there is no satisfactory curative therapy. Liver transplantation remains the treatment of choice for patients with end-stage chronic liver disease.

1.5.21

Haemochromatosis

The term "haemochromatosis" is defined as the progressive deposition of iron in the parenchymal cells of many organs leading to cell damage and functional insufficiency. In the liver parenchymal iron deposition leads to fibrosis and cirrhosis. A group of disorders gives rise to the clinicopathologic syndrome of haemochromatosis (*Table 42*).

EPIDEMIOLOGY AND PATHOGENESIS

The mechanisms by which iron causes tissue damage are unknown. Instability of lysosomal membranes due to

Notes

Table 42 Iron overload conditions

Genetic haemochromatosis (primary, idiopathic)
Secondary haemochromatosis
Anaemia, including ineffective erythropoiesis/haemolysis (e.g. thalassaemia and sideroblastic anaemia)
Liver disease with secondary iron overload (e.g. alcohol, porphyria cutanea tarda, portacaval shunt)
Excessive iron ingestion or absorption (e.g. Bantu siderosis, excess medicinal iron ingestion)

increased haemosiderin deposition, intracellular membrane damage caused by peroxidase degradation of membrane lipids, and a direct fibrogenic effect of iron are possible mechanisms. These are not mutually exclusive and disease may well result from a combination.

Genetic haemochromatosis (primary or idiopathic haemochromatosis)

This is a recessively inherited condition in which there is inappropriate absorption of iron by the duodenal mucosa. This raises serum iron and decreases serum transferrin concentrations, but increases transferrin saturation. Tissue iron accumulation is very slow, so disease aften presents after the age of 40 years in men when iron stores are usually greater than 20 g (compared with a normal value of 1 g). Physiologic iron loss through menstruation and pregnancy delays presentation in women. The gene frequency can be as high as 1 in 20 in some Western populations, with a frequency of homozygosity of 1 in 300. The gene for haemochroma-

Notes

tosis is on chromosome 6p in close association with the histocompatibility antigen HLA-A3 and also HLA-B7 and HLA-B14. Recently the defect has been localized to a mutation of a major histocompatibility complex (MHC) class I molecule termed HLA-H. This mutation probably accounts for more than 80% of patients with genetic haemochromatosis.

PRESENTATION

The clinical manifestations of genetic haemochromatosis in symptomatic patients are shown in *Table 43*. The pigmentation is due to melanin stimulated by iron deposition in the skin. Two thirds develop an arthropathy of the small joints of the hands, wrists, and knees related to the deposition of crystals – "pseudogout". Some carbohydrate intolerance is seen in about 90% but

Table 43 Clinical features in symptomatic patients with genetic haemochromatosis

Clinical feature	Approximate proportion affected (%)
Skin pigmentation (greyish-brown)	80
Early menopause or loss of libido	80
Malaise, weight loss, abdominal pain	70
Hepatomegaly	70
Diabetes mellitus	50–60
Arthropathy (especially 2nd/3rd metacarpophalangeal joints)/ pseudogout	50
Congestive cardiac failure	15

Notes

only about half require insulin. Many patients, however, are asymptomatic and are detected on the basis of biochemical screening.

INVESTIGATIONS

1.5

Transferrin saturation and serum ferritin concentration are useful screening tests and, if normal (ferritin 30–350 $\mu g\,l^{-1}$ in men and 20–150 $\mu g\,l^{-1}$ in women), then significant iron overload is excluded. The serum ferritin level reflects the magnitude of iron stores in the body. In addition to it being raised in genetic haemochromatosis, it can be increased in liver disease, inflammation, leukemia, lymphoma, cancer and infections. In alcoholic liver disease the ferritin concentration is often raised (usually less than 1000 $\mu g\,l^{-1}$) because of hepatic inflammation/necrosis or alcohol consumption *per se*. Serum iron level (normal 10–30 $\mu m\,l^{-1}$) is usually raised in genetic haemochromatosis, but is not specific. The iron-binding capacity of transferrin (percentage transferrin saturation) is a more reliable indicator. A transferrin saturation of greater than 55% is more sensitive and specific for genetic haemochromatosis than an increased ferritin concentration. The transferrin saturation may be raised in severe alcohol-related liver disease because of decreased hepatic synthesis of transferrin.

Liver histopathology and chemical analysis of hepatic iron concentration usually distinguishes genetic haemochromatosis from other conditions. Slight to moderate levels of stainable iron may be seen with heavy alcohol consumption or in elderly heterozygotes for the haemochromatosis gene. In homozygous haemochromatosis

Notes

there is markedly increased stainable iron, unless the subject is young or there has been regular blood loss (therapeutic phlebotomy, menstruation, gastrointestinal blood loss). The hepatic iron index (hepatic iron concentration ($\mu mol\,g^{-1}$ dry weight) divided by age in years) allows for variation in age and is a better discriminator than the hepatic iron concentration alone.

An hepatic iron index greater than 2 is highly suggestive of genetic haemochromatosis. Genetic testing and screening will be possible in the near future.

MANAGEMENT

Excess iron is removed by phlebotomy in patients with genetic haemochromatosis. Regular weekly venesection removing 500 ml blood (equivalent to 250 mg iron) is performed until iron stores are normalized, usually over 1–2 years. In contrast, chelation therapy removes only 10–20 mg iron per day. Weekly phlebotomy is continued until the serum ferritin level reaches 10 $mg\,l^{-1}$ or the transferrin saturation normalizes or the haemoglobin level drops to 10.5 $g\,dl^{-1}$ and fails to rise indicating depletion of iron stores. Thereafter, phlebotomy every 3 months is usually required long-term. Phlebotomy produces a rapid improvement in lethargy and malaise but does not affect arthropathy or diabetes. Venesection in cirrhotic patients improves the 5-year survival rate markedly, from 18 to 80% by reducing deaths from hepatic failure, variceal bleeding, and cardiac failure. It does not prevent the development in cirrhotic patients of primary liver cell cancer, which may occur up to 15 years after iron depletion. In patients who progress to liver

Notes

transplantation, post-transplant survival may be reduced by cardiac events, especially arrhythmias or heart failure. These complications may be related to inadequate pretransplant de-ironing. First-degree relatives of patients with proven genetic haemochromatosis should be screened so that disease may be detected and treated at an early stage.

1.5.22

α_1-Antitrypsin Deficiency

EPIDEMIOLOGY AND PATHOGENESIS

The protease inhibitor α_1-antitrypsin is synthesized in the endoplasmic reticulum of the liver and accounts for approximately 80–90% of the serum α_1 globulin. Classic α_1-antitrypsin deficiency (Pi (protein inhibitor) ZZ phenotype) is a codominantly inherited disease that is associated with pulmonary emphysema and liver disease. α_1-antitrypsin levels are usually 10–15% of normal.

A defect in transport out of the hepatocyte with deposition of excess α_1 trypsin globules within the liver cells probably causes liver disease. The incidence of hepatic injury is high during the first year of life (about 75%) and steadily decreases until adulthood. Less than 5% of affected children will need liver transplantation. In adults, only 10–20% of α_1-antitrypsin-deficient homozygotes develop significant liver dysfunction. Males are twice as likely to develop liver disease as females.

Notes

Although obstructive lung disease is the predominant disease manifestation of homozygous α_1-antitrypsin deficiency, in those with liver disease it is often only mild or subclinical.

It is unclear whether heterozygotes (Pi MZ, Pi SZ) are more likely to develop liver disease than those with a normal phenotype (Pi MM). A single amino acid replacement of glutamic acid at positions 264 and 342 of the α_1-antitrypsin polypeptide results in the S and Z variants respectively.

PRESENTATION

The majority of patients present with hepatic or cholestatic jaundice within the first 4 months of life. If the period of neonatal jaundice is survived then the liver disease may go into remission for many years, presenting at a later stage as cirrhosis and its complications.

INVESTIGATIONS

The diagnosis may be suspected by a low serum α_1-antitrypsin level in a patient with chronic liver disease. Heterozygotes with liver disease or inflammation may have normal levels. Phenotyping may be done by isoelectric focusing in which the proteins are divided into medium (M), slow (S), or very slow (Z) bands by their electrophoretic characteristics. Liver histology confirms globules of α_1-antitrypsin (by immunoperoxidase stain) in the periportal regions. Patients who are heterozygous for the Z phenotype, especially Pi MZ, can also have extensive α_1-antitrypsin deposition.

Notes

MANAGEMENT

There is no specific treatment for α_1-antitrypsin-deficiency liver disease. For decompensated chronic liver disease, hepatic transplantation may be undertaken if not contraindicated by serious pulmonary disease. After transplantation the α_1-antitrypsin phenotype of the donor predominates.

1.5.23

Wilson's Disease (Hepatolenticular Degeneration)

Wilson's disease is a rare inborn error of copper metabolism characterized by excessive amounts of copper in various organs producing cirrhosis of the liver, bilateral degeneration of the basal ganglia of the brain, and greenish-brown pigmented rings in the periphery of the cornea (Kayser–Fleischer rings). Other organs, particularly the kidney, are also affected.

EPIDEMIOLOGY AND PATHOGENESIS

Inheritance is autosomal recessive and produces a low plasma level of ceruloplasmin, the copper transport protein, and also copper. Biliary copper excretion is low but urinary copper excretion is characteristically increased. The gene has been localized to chromosome 13q14.3 which codes for a copper-transporting P-type ATPase protein. Over 30 mutations have been identified which result in defective biliary excretion of copper and

Notes

reduced incorporation of copper into ceruloplasmin. The disease is found worldwide. The prevalence is about 1 in 30 000 with a carrier frequency of about 1 in 90.

PRESENTATION

In children, liver disease predominates, whereas adults over the age of 20 years usually have neurologic symptoms. The two types may overlap. Most patients are diagnosed between the ages of 5 and 30 years. Wilson's disease may present as *acute hepatitis, fulminant hepatitis, chronic active hepatitis* or insidiously as *cirrhosis*. The fulminant hepatitis is characterized by a haemolytic anaemia produced by a sudden influx of copper from dying hepatocytes into the serum. The neurologic problems are tremour, dysarthria, involuntary movements, and a progressive deterioration in mental function. Psychiatric disease, including psychosis, can be a clinical feature.

Renal tubular damage, due to copper deposits, may be present with glycosuria, phosphaturia, and uricosuria. Renal tubular acidosis can also occur.

INVESTIGATIONS

Copper deposition in Descemet's membrane results in a corneal crescent or ring (Kayser–Fleischer rings); these are best demonstrated by slit-lamp examination. Kayser–Fleischer rings are present in virtually all patients with cerebral manifestations of Wilson's disease. They are less frequent, however, in those with liver disease. They may also be rarely seen in secondary copper overload, such as in primary biliary cirrhosis.

Notes

Serum ceruloplasmin and copper levels are usually reduced but can be normal in a minority of cases. A low normal ceruloplasmin in Wilson's disease (about 15% of patients with symptomatic liver disease) may be due to the effect of hepatic inflammation on this acute phase reactant. The 24-hour urinary copper excretion is nearly always increased (more than 80 μg or 1.25 μmol per day). A rate greater than 200 μg per day has been considered diagnostic; heterozygotes rarely excrete more than 100 μg per day. In patients with equivocal urinary copper excretion a "penicillamine challenge test" can be undertaken. Patients are given 250 μg of penicillamine every 6 hours for 48 hours. Urinary copper excretion in the latter 24 hours is up to 800 μg in normals, and greater than 1000 μg in those with Wilson's disease; more than 2000 μg a day is considered diagnostic, and up to 1500 μg daily can occur in heterozygotes.

Hepatic histology is nondiagnostic showing anything from periportal inflammation and fibrosis through submassive necrosis to a macronodular cirrhosis. Steatosis and periportal Mallory bodies are a frequent feature. Excess copper may be seen with special stains, although this is unreliable. Hepatic copper concentration can be measured directly by neutron activation. In untreated Wilson's disease the hepatic copper concentration is usually in excess of 250 μg per g dry weight (normal value less than 50 μg per g dry weight). The occasional patient may have a hepatic copper concentration less than 250 $\mu g\, g^{-1}$, which may make distinction from the heterozygous state difficult, especially in the young. High hepatic copper levels are also found in secondary causes of copper overload, such as long-standing cholestasis.

Notes

MANAGEMENT

Long-term use of the chelating agent penicillamine is effective, removing tissue copper and increasing urinary copper excretion, and leading to a slow progressive clinical and biochemical improvement. Symptomatic neurologic damage is usually permanent. The initial dose of penicillamine in an adolescent or an adult is 500 mg orally three times a day about 20 min before meals (children: 25 $mg\,kg^{-1}$ total daily dosage). If necessary the dose can be increased to 2–3 g per day. If the patient is presymptomatic or symptoms have been controlled for at least 1 year and copper stores depleted, the dose may be reduced to 0.75^{-1} g per day. Treatment is monitored by 24-hour urinary copper excretion and liver biopsy. Side-effects of penicillamine are unusual but include rashes, leucopenia, proteinuria, and aplastic anaemia. If reactions are not manageable by dose reduction, cessation of penicillamine and use of the orally active chelating agent trientine dihydrochloride (initially 600 mg three times a day, then twice a day as per penicillamine) is appropriate. Penicillamine may cause pyridoxine deficiency. A dose of 50 mg *pyridoxine* once per week will prevent this. Zinc reduces copper absorption and may be a useful adjunct to penicillamine. It is given as zinc sulphate 50 mg three times a day before food.

Liver transplantation is curative and may be indicated in patients with fulminant hepatic failure or severe irreversible liver disease. Liver transplantation may also be appropriate in patients with progressive neurologic disease despite adequate medical therapy, even if there is only minimal or well-compensated liver disease, because substantial improvements in neurologic function usually occur following transplant.

Biochemical and ophthalmologic screening of relatives is vital to discover asymptomatic subjects, as disease progression can be prevented by intervention with penicillamine therapy. It is now also possible to undertake genetic screening for common mutations, and in addition to type several markers flanking the gene for Wilson's disease.

1.5.24

Fibropolycystic Diseases

EPIDEMIOLOGY AND PATHOGENESIS

The increased and widened use of imaging techniques such as ultrasonography and computed tomography has led to an increasing diagnosis of cystic lesions of the hepatobiliary system. These imaging techniques have shown that the fibrocystic diseases are all part of the same disease spectrum and can exist in various combinations. Fibrocystic disease of the kidneys is associated with all these conditions to a variable degree. Cancer, particularly biliary, can complicate all types of polycystic disease.

Childhood fibropolycystic disease

Childhood fibropolycystic disease is classified into perinatal, neonatal, infantile, and juvenile. All forms

Notes

are autosomal recessively inherited. The extent of renal involvement determines the prognosis. In the *perinatal* type there are huge renal masses; death, if not stillborn, usually occurs within a few weeks of delivery. The *neonatal* type is associated primarily with renal failure and hypertension; portal fibrosis and cystic dilatation of the bile ducts is common, and cholangitis is a frequent complication. In the *infantile* group there is either chronic renal failure or increasing portal hypertension; portal fibrosis is moderate. The *juvenile* group includes children aged 1–5 years who present with portal hypertension. There are renal cysts. Hepatic cysts are rare but there are irregularly dilated bile ducts and hepatic fibrosis.

Adult fibropolycystic disease

In adult fibropolycystic disease the cysts arise from defective development of the intrahepatic bile ducts in the portal tracts. The condition is autosomal dominant and frequently associated with polycystic kidneys. The abnormal gene is on the short arm of chromosome 16. The mode of presentation depends on the number and size of the cysts. On many occasions liver lesions in patients are diagnosed either on routine ultrasonography or at autopsy. Symptomatic patients present in middle age with abdominal pain and distension. Liver function is normal as the hepatocytes are not involved and the development of complications, such as ascites, jaundice, and oesophageal varices, is rare. The most common hepatic problem is infection of liver cysts, with cholangiocarcinoma the second most common.

Notes

Congenital hepatic fibrosis

Congenital hepatic fibrosis is an autosomal recessive condition in which normal hepatic lobules are surrounded and divided by densely collagenous fibrous bands arising from portal tracts. There may be associated dilatation of intrahepatic and extrahepatic ducts. The condition occurs predominantly in children and adolescents.

Some patients may have cystic kidneys similar to adult polycystic disease. However, the more common kidney disease is medullary tubular ectasia in which there is cystic dilatation of tubules.

Liver function is well maintained for many years but portal hypertension is common. Patients may present with variceal haemorrhage or with the discovery of hepatosplenomegaly. Recurrent cholangitis can also be a feature. Diagnosis is established by hepatic biopsy and the condition must be distinguished from cirrhosis, which has a worse prognosis.

Congenital intrahepatic biliary dilatation (Caroli's disease)

This rare condition is characterized by multiple saccular dilatations of the intrahepatic bile ducts. The cystic dilatations are 1.0–4.5 cm in diameter. They are part of the main duct system and may be separated by essentially normal duct. Recurrent cholangitis, abscess formation, septicemia, intrahepatic stones, and amyloidosis are all complications. The inheritance is autosomal recessive. Caroli's disease can be associated with

Notes

congenital hepatic fibrosis (Caroli's "syndrome") and rarely with other fibropolycystic diseases.

PRESENTATION

In fibropolycystic disease liver function is initially generally good, although portal hypertension develops and complications can ensue. Patients may present with bleeding or hepatosplenomegaly. Biliary dilatation usually presents with pain, fever, and jaundice due to infection.

INVESTIGATIONS

Liver function tests are usually normal, except for moderately increased concentrations of alkaline phosphatase and γ-glutamyl transpeptidase. Ultrasonography and cholangiography are the key diagnostic tools. Liver biopsy may be necessary to confirm hepatic fibrosis and exclude alternative diagnoses. Blood cultures are appropriate if sepsis is suspected.

MANAGEMENT

Treatment is primarily for the complications of portal hypertension, especially variceal haemorrhage (see *1.5.1 Variceal Bleeding*) and recurrent biliary sepsis. The management of acute episodes of bacterial cholangitis is with appropriate antibiotics. The occurrence of recurrent episodes also may be reduced by long-term periodic use of antibiotics, such as oral trimethoprim or a cephalosporin. Common duct stones, which may be a feature of Caroli's disease, can be removed endoscopically; however,

Notes

recurrent sepsis usually occurs because of intrahepatic stones and strictures. The same problem can occur with surgical drainage. However, surgical resection of an affected area may be possible. In patients with biliary stones, ursodeoxycholic acid (10–15 mg per kg body weight orally per day in divided doses) may be beneficial. In diffuse disease with severe recurrent complications, liver transplantation is a consideration.

1.5.25

Overview of Hepatic Tumours

The primary tumours that arise in the hepatobiliary system are shown in *Table 44*. The commonest liver tumours, however, are secondary deposits.

1.5.26

Hepatocellular Carcinoma (Hepatoma)

EPIDEMIOLOGY AND PATHOGENESIS

The frequency of hepatocellular carcinoma varies geographically being relatively rare in the West but particularly frequent in Asia and Africa. There is a strong association with hepatitis B infection although the mechanism by which hepatitis B virus initiates carcinogenesis is still uncertain (see *1.5.9 Hepatitis B*). The risk of developing hepatocellular cancer is 400 times greater in patients in the East who are positive for hepatitis B surface

Notes

Table 44 Tumours affecting the hepatobiliary system

	Benign	**Malignant**
Biliary	Adenoma Cystadenoma Papillomatosis Fibroma	Cholangiocarcinoma Carcinoma of the gallbladder Cystadenocarcinoma
Hepatic	Adenoma Haemangioma	Hepatocellular carcinoma Fibrolamellar carcinoma Haemangiosarcoma Sarcoma Mixed (hepatobiliary carcinoma)
Hepatic pseudotumour	Cysts Focal nodular hyperplasia Pseudolipoma	

antigen (HBsAg), especially those who have developed cirrhosis. Hepatitis C has also been linked directly to the development of primary liver cancer (see *1.5.11 Hepatitis C*). The male : female ratio is about 6 : 1. Primary liver cancer may also complicate other forms of cirrhosis, particularly haemochromatosis and alcoholic cirrhosis. Other carcinogens have also been implicated, particularly aflatoxins (which are produced by *Aspergillus flavus* and contaminated groundnuts or by grain stored under tropical conditions) and anabolic steroids.

Hepatocellular carcinoma may be single or multifocal. The tumour cells resemble normal liver and may secrete bile. The tumour commonly metastasizes to involve regional and distant lymph nodes, peritoneum, lung, and bones.

Notes

PRESENTATION

There are no symptoms or signs that are pathognomonic of hepatocellular carcinoma, and diagnosis is usually late except in cases detected by screening. In Western countries, hepatoma should be considered in patients with known cirrhosis who deteriorate or develop a mass in the right upper quadrant. Features include weight loss, malaise, unexplained fever, right upper quadrant pain, ascites, and jaundice. Examination may reveal a large tender liver, often with an arterial bruit. In tropical Africa, hepatoma tends to have a fulminating course that mimics liver abscess; patients are usually young adults with cirrhosis being noted at the same time. In the Far East the presentation is somewhere between the above.

Paraneoplastic syndromes that may be associated with hepatoma include hypoglycemia, hypercalcemia, erythrocytosis, hypercholesterolemia, and sexual changes such as gynecomastia and feminization.

INVESTIGATIONS

Measurement of α-foetoprotein levels is useful in diagnosis and to follow response to treatment, but in caucasian patients it is not raised in 30% of cases. Modest increases also occur with hepatocyte regeneration, especially after hepatic necrosis but also with chronic hepatitis and cirrhosis. These rises are often related to transaminase activity and are transient or episodic.

Hepatomas are localized by ultrasonography, and computed tomography is used particularly to demonstrate

Notes

the extent of hepatic involvement. On ultrasonography small hepatomas may be hypoechoic or have a hypoechoic rim, or they may be hyperechoic (resembling a small haemangioma); larger hepatomas can also be either hypoechoic, hyperechoic, or mixed with coexistent cirrhotic features. On CT the hepatoma is usually hypodense (around 10% isodense), and enhances rapidly and uniformly with dynamic scanning. Angiography is frequently used for diagnosis, localization, and to determine the extent of the tumour before possible surgical resection. In Asia, screening programs have resulted in increasing numbers of patients being diagnosed with tumours less than 2 cm in diameter.

Although the diagnosis can be confirmed by liver biopsy, usually performed under ultrasonographic guidance, biopsy should be avoided if the tumour is suitable for hepatic resection. Biopsy of the normal appearing liver, however, is useful in assessing the suitability of resection versus transplantation.

MANAGEMENT

Small tumours may be resected surgically or liver transplantation may be performed. Overall, the resectability rate is low, however. Chemotherapy with doxorubicin is used but the prognosis is poor and the tumours are not radiosensitive. Injection with absolute ethanol or arterial embolization are approaches that may reduce tumour growth. The survival of patients with tumours greater than 2 cm is rarely more than 1 year.

Notes

Screening for hepatocellular carcinoma

Screening for hepatocellular carcinoma is appropriate for people at high risk. This includes those with hepatitis B or hepatitis C cirrhosis, especially if aged over 40 years, of Asian or African background, or with a family history of hepatocellular carcinoma. Hepatic ultrasonography and estimation of serum α-foetoprotein levels at 3–6-month intervals is recommended.

1.5.27

Cholangiocarcinoma

EPIDEMIOLOGY AND PATHOGENESIS

The frequency of carcinoma of the bile ducts (cholangiocarcinoma), although less than that of hepatoma, is increasing. The cancer is usually an adenocarcinoma and is most frequently extrahepatic rather than intrahepatic. Bile duct cancer is associated with primary sclerosing cholangitis (see *1.5.20*), congenital fibropolycystic disease (see *1.5.24*), choledochal cysts, and biliary cirrhosis secondary to biliary atresia. The highest incidence of cholangiocarcinoma is in the Far East where it is associated with infestation with the liver flukes *Clonorchis sinensis* and *Opisthorchis viverrini*.

PRESENTATION

Malaise, weight loss, right upper quadrant pain and a progressive deepening jaundice are usual. There may be

Notes

associated ascending cholangitis or haemobilia. In intrahepatic cholangiocarcinoma, however, jaundice is rare.

INVESTIGATIONS

Blood tests show cholestasis (raised alkaline phosphatase and γ-glutamyl transpeptidase levels), and ultrasonography and computed tomography may be helpful. Cholangiography, either endoscopically (by means of endoscopic retrograde cholangiopancreatography (ERCP)), percutaneously, or with magnetic resonance imaging, is the mainstay of diagnosis.

MANAGEMENT

Surgical resection of a cholangiocarcinoma is possible in only 20% or less of cases. Palliation can be performed by the endoscopic or transhepatic insertion of a biliary prosthesis. Internal radiotherapy using Iridium-192 wires has also been advocated. Adjuvant chemotherapy has not been demonstrated to be of benefit. The prognosis depends on age and the extent of tumour. Half of the patients die within 1 year of diagnosis.

1.5.28

Carcinoma of the Gallbladder

EPIDEMIOLOGY AND PATHOGENESIS

Carcinoma of the gallbladder is the fifth most common gastrointestinal cancer. It has the worst prognosis,

Notes

however, because the cancer is usually well advanced before it becomes symptomatic. Gallbladder cancer occurs most commonly in elderly women and is frequently associated with gallstones.

PRESENTATION

Patients present with weight loss, right upper quadrant pain, and jaundice, and a mass is frequently palpable in the right upper quadrant. Jaundice is usually the result of tumour involvement of the common bile duct.

INVESTIGATIONS

Ultrasonography and computed tomography are the main initial investigations. Cholangiography, either endoscopically (ERCP), percutaneously, or with magnetic resonance imaging, is also frequently helpful.

MANAGEMENT

Cholecystectomy should be performed in patients in whom the cancer has not metastasized, although this is very unusual and the mean length of survival from diagnosis is approximately 6 months. Extensive hepatic resection has not been demonstrated to improve survival rates. Endoscopic or transhepatic insertion of a biliary stent may be necessary if the common bile duct is involved.

Notes

1.5.29

Hepatic Adenoma

Hepatic adenomas are benign tumours associated with oestrogen-containing oral contraceptives and pregnancy. They can, however, be difficult to distinguish from hepatocellular carcinoma. Hepatic adenomas are usually diagnosed in women aged between 15 and 45 years. They are usually asymptomatic and found coincidentally. However, patients may present with abdominal pain (from intratumoural haemorrhage), an abdominal mass, or shock from intraperitoneal bleeding. Ultrasonography and computed tomography show a solid tumour. Hepatic angiography may demonstrate a nourishing artery at the periphery of the tumour with branches penetrating it. Withdrawal of oestrogen therapy is important. Surgical resection should be considered if there is no reduction in size with cessation of contraceptives.

1.5.30

Focal Nodular Hyperplasia

Focal nodular hyperplasia is a benign tumour-like lesion that occurs in both sexes and at any age but is most common in young women. Most are discovered incidentally. Some cause symptoms such as awareness of an abdominal mass or pain. Rupture with acute haemoperitoneum is a rare occurrence. Although not caused by oestrogen-containing oral contraceptives, these drugs and pregnancy can have a trophic effect with an increase in vascularity and a predisposition to rupture. Imaging

Notes

techniques are the main investigation, although focal nodular hyperplasia can be difficult to distinguish from hepatic adenoma. A common characteristic feature on computed tomography is a hypodense central zone due to a fibrous stellate central scar. On angiography an artery may be demonstrated to penetrate the tumour with several branches. Most patients are treated conservatively although oestrogen therapy should be withdrawn. Surgery may be necessary if there are symptoms or the diagnosis is doubtful.

1.5.31

Gallstones

EPIDEMIOLOGY AND PATHOGENESIS

Approximately 10–20% of the population in the Western world develop gallstones. There are three major types (*Table 45*).

Cholesterol gallstones

Cholesterol stones account for nearly 80% of gallstones occurring in the Western hemisphere. These stones contain at least 50% by weight of cholesterol monohydrate. Solitary gallstones are usually pure cholesterol and multiple stones are usually of mixed composition. Cholesterol gallstones are associated with increasing age, female sex, and obesity (*Table 46*). In normal subjects insoluble cholesterol is kept in solution by the formation of micelles which are composed of cholesterol, bile salts,

Notes

Table 45 Classification and characteristics of gallstone types

Type	Cholesterol	Black	Brown
Major constituents	Cholesterol Bile pigments Calcium salts Mucoprotein matrix	Calcium bilirubinate (polymerized)	Calcium bilirubinate (precipitated salt) Calcium palmitate Cholesterol
Consistency	Crystalline	Hard	Soft, friable
Location	Gallbladder and bile ducts	Gallbladder	Intrahepatic and extrahepatic bile ducts
Proportion radio-opaque (%)	15	60	0

Table 46 Risk factors for cholesterol stones

Established	Possible
Female sex	Family history of gallstones
Obesity	Oral contraceptives
Age	Pregnancy
Crash dieting	Diabetes mellitus
Terminal ileal disease	High polyunsaturated fat diet
Cystic fibrosis	
High spinal injury	
Clofibrate therapy	

and phospholipid. People who develop cholesterol gallstones secrete supersaturated bile in which there is an excess of cholesterol, relative to bile salts and

Notes

phosopholipids. This is usually due to a diminished hepatic secretion of bile acids, secondary to a reduced total body pool of bile acids. Secretion of nucleating factors that predispose to cholesterol precipitation and abnormal gallbladder function are also pathogenic features.

Pigment gallstones

Pigment stones account for about 20% of gallstones, although they are more common in some Asian countries. Black stones are frequently found in patients with chronic haemolytic anaemia or cirrhosis. Brown stones are associated with infections in the biliary tract, notably parasitic infestations such as *Clonorchis sinensis* and *Ascaris lumbricoides* in the Far East.

PRESENTATION

In most patients gallstones remain in the gallbladder where they are symptomless (silent gallstones). Symptoms develop when stones migrate into the neck of the gallbladder or into the common bile duct. A gallstone impacting in the neck of the gallbladder or the cystic duct causes either biliary colic or cholecystitis. Biliary colic can be defined as a steady epigastric and/or right hypochondrial pain that usually lasts more than 15–30 min and is not relieved by defaecation or the passing of flatus. Gallstones that pass into the common bile duct may pass uneventfully into the duodenum or remain silently in the common duct. Frequently such stones cause biliary obstruction giving biliary colic and/or cholestatic

Notes

jaundice. Bacterial infection may follow and produce cholangitis with fever, rigours, and abdominal pain. Rarely, an internal biliary fistula can arise from the migration of a gallstone from the inflamed gallbladder into an adjacent viscus. The stone may be passed uneventfully in the faeces or impact at the ileocecal valve causing gallstone ileus.

MANAGEMENT

Only a minority of patients with silent gallstones will develop symptoms during the rest of their lives, and asymptomatic gallstones require no treatment. Various options are available.

Medical treatment

Noncalcified cholesterol gallstones can be dissolved by oral bile acid therapy with either chenodeoxycholic acid and/or *ursodeoxycholic acid* (see 2.3.2). Approximately 60% of gallstones will dissolve or partially dissolve after 2 years of treatment. Patients who are suitable for this treatment are those with floating small cholesterol gallstones in a functioning gallbladder. Dissolution rates are poor in obese patients. Chenodeoxycholic acid produces an increase in serum levels of transaminases and diarrhoea. Ursodeoxycholic acid may cause calcification of gallstones. Side-effects can be reduced by combination therapy with both agents using lower doses (chenodeoxycholic acid 7.5 mg per kg daily and ursodeoxycholic acid 5 mg per kg daily).

Notes

Chemical dissolution

Noncalcified cholesterol gallstones can be dissolved by passing a pigtail catheter into the gallbladder via a percutaneous transhepatic route under fluoroscopic or ultrasonographic guidance and infusing methyltertbutyl ether (MTBE). This is a powerful chemical solvent which rapidly dissolves the gallstones. It probably should be attempted only if the cystic duct is patent, and is recommended for specialist use only.

Extracorporeal shockwave lithotripsy (ESWL)

Pulsed shockwaves are focused by ultrasound on to stones within the gallbladder until the stone(s) shatter. It is suitable for one or two cholesterol gallstones in a functioning gallbladder. Adjuvant therapy with chenodeoxycholic acid and ursodeoxycholic acid is begun 2 weeks before lithotripsy, and is continued for 2 months following disappearance of gallstones on ultrasonography, so that the fragments are dissolved. Side-effects are few, but include acute pancreatitis.

Percutaneous cholecystolithotomy

This technique involves gallbladder puncture under radiologic control via a subhepatic transperitoneal approach. A wide-bore (22–26 Fr) tube is inserted to allow the use of endoscopes, grasping forceps, Dormier baskets, and contact lithotripsy probes for removal or fragmentation of gallstones. The procedure is done under general anaesthesia but has fewer perioperative risks than open abdominal cholecystectomy. The gallbladder

Notes

remains *in situ* and stone recurrence is a significant risk.

Cholecystectomy

This surgical procedure remains a safe procedure with a low morbidity and mortality rate of less than 1% in skilled hands. The common bile duct should be explored in patients with a history of jaundice or biliary colic. Laparoscopic cholecystectomy has recently been introduced and in skilled hands reduces morbidity and hospital stay. Cholecystectomy remains the main mode of treatment for symptomatic gallstones.

1.5.32

Cholecystitis

EPIDEMIOLOGY AND PATHOGENESIS

In the majority of patients with acute cholecystitis the cystic duct is obstructed by a stone producing distension and inflammation of the gallbladder wall. The bile is usually infected with enteric organisms. The organisms involved are predominantly aerobic such as *Escherichia coli, Klebsiella* species, and less commonly *Enterococcus faecalis*. In extreme cases the rise in gallbladder pressure causes infarction and gangrene. The gallbladder may be distended by pus (empyema). A mucocele occurs when the inflammation is mild and the obstructed gallbladder becomes distended with mucus.

About 10% of gallbladders removed for "acute" cholecystitis do not contain gallstones but are associated

Notes

with burns or severe sepsis. It is likely that ischaemia plays an important role, leading to superadded infection and sepsis. This may lead to gangrene and perforation of the gallbladder. The mortality rate from acute acalculous cholecystitis is high.

Chronic cholecystitis can follow an acute attack but more usually it has an insidious onset. The gallbladder is usually thickened but contracted and contains gallstones. Histologically there is marked fibrosis and muscular hypertrophy of the gallbladder wall.

PRESENTATION

Cholecystitis can occur acutely at any age, although classically it occurs in obese women of childbearing age. In acute cholecystitis the features may be that of an "acute abdomen". Symptoms are of right upper quadrant and epigastric pain which may radiate to the shoulder and back. Nausea and vomiting may occur. Fever and right hypochondrial tenderness, guarding, and rebound may be characteristic. The presence of jaundice usually suggests obstruction to the common bile duct. In chronic cholecystitis the symptoms tend to be vague and nonspecific, and clinical signs are usually absent. Pain or discomfort occurs in the right upper quadrant, especially after a heavy meal. It can also radiate to the shoulder and back. Less specific symptoms include bloating and abdominal distension.

INVESTIGATIONS

Laboratory findings that may be present include a raised white blood count due to a polymorph leucocytosis, and

Notes

a mild increase in the levels of bilirubin, aspartate aminotransferase (ASAT), and alkaline phosphatase. Ultrasonography examination is particularly helpful and may show a thickened gallbladder wall and the presence of gallstones. If there is diagnostic doubt then an iminodiacetic acid (HIDA) scintiscan can be performed. In patients with acute cholecystitis no filling of the gallbladder or cystic duct is observed. The sensitivity of this investigation is greater than 90% in acute disease.

MANAGEMENT

Management depends on severity but general measures for acute cholecystitis include bedrest and pain relief with either opiates, such as pethidine, or a nonsteroidal analgesic, such as diclofenac. Patients in severe pain with vomiting should receive intravenous fluids, and complications such as peritonitis are an indication for acute surgery.

Antibiotics should be given to cover infections from enteric organisms. Suitable antimicrobial therapy is (amoxy)ampicillin 1 g intravenously 6 hourly and gentamicin 5–7 $mg\,kg^{-1}day^{-1}$ intravenously, once daily. If either antibiotic is contraindicated then an alternative is cefotaxime 1 g intravenously 8 hourly or ceftriaxone 1 g intravenously, once daily. Cephalosporins, however, are inactive against *Enterococcus faecalis.*

Traditional practice has been to allow the inflammation to settle and to perform cholecystectomy 6–8 weeks later. Now the preferred practice is to undertake cholecystectomy within a few days of the acute attack. This is not associated with greater morbidity or mortality. If surgery is delayed there is the risk of a further attack of acute cholecystitis or other complications of gallstone disease.

In chronic cholecystitis, the traditional conservative treatment has been a low fat diet. However, there may be ongoing symptoms, and there is also a risk of acute cholecystitis. Thus elective cholecystectomy should be recommended.

1.5.33

Common Bile Duct Stones

EPIDEMIOLOGY AND PATHOGENESIS

Stones in the common bile duct arise in two ways. In most cases stones are passed from the gallbladder. The epidemiology and pathogenesis of such stones covered in *Section 1.5.31*. Other stones, predominantly brown pigment, arise *de novo* in the common bile duct, often secondary to partial biliary obstruction from a variety of causes, such as sclerosing cholangitis and traumatic strictures.

PRESENTATION

Common duct stones may be asymptomatic, discovered only on routine screening. In the elderly patient they should be remembered as a cause of unexplained mental and physical debility. Stones may give rise to any one or all of the symptoms of abdominal pain, jaundice, rigours, and fever. The abdominal pain is usually centred in the right upper quadrant but may occur in the epigastrium

Notes

and lower chest. Stools become pale and the urine is dark. The degree of jaundice is variable and may be intermittent, particularly when the stone acts as a ball valve at the lower end of the common bile duct. In addition, stones impacted in the ampulla of Vater may give rise to acute pancreatitis. Common duct stones are usually associated with infected bile which can result in systemic sepsis (see *1.5.34 Acute Cholangitis*).

INVESTIGATIONS

A polymorph leucocytosis is expected and blood cultures may reveal enteric organisms such as *Escherichia coli*. Liver function tests show a cholestatic pattern with a raised level of alkaline phosphatase and bilirubin, and a variable rise in aspartate aminotransaminase (AST). There is no derangement in clotting unless the obstruction is complete and prolonged. Ultrasonography usually reveals a dilated ductal system but may not demonstrate a stone. ERCP confirms the presence of stones and may enable their removal.

MANAGEMENT

The management of common bile duct stones depends on the clinical situation. Episodes associated with acute cholangitis are treated with antibiotics (see *1.5.34 Acute Cholangitis*) and then the stones are removed either by the endoscopic route or at surgery. Different options are discussed further below.

Notes

Chemical dissolution

Some stones that have passed out of the gallbladder into the bile ducts can be dissolved using infusing methyl-tertbutyl ether (MTBE) administered through a naso-biliary catheter inserted at ERCP. The technique is less successful than that used for gallbladder stones but a 50% success rate is claimed. The procedure is labour intensive.

Extracorporeal shockwave lithotripsy

This technique (see *1.5.31 Gallstones*) has been increasingly employed for treatment of large common bile duct stones that cannot be removed via endoscopy.

Endoscopic therapy

Gallstones may be removed following a sphincterotomy using a Dormier basket or balloon catheter. This technique is employed in the elderly or those unfit for surgery, particularly when the gallbladder has been removed previously. Complications of this technique include haemorrhage in approximately 5% of cases and acute pancreatitis.

Surgery

In young fit patients cholecystectomy and exploration of the common bile duct is carried out. In older patients endoscopic therapy is preferred to limit morbidity.

Notes

1.5.34

Acute Cholangitis

EPIDEMIOLOGY AND PATHOGENESIS

Acute cholangitis is defined as bacterial infection of the bile duct excluding the gallbladder. The commonest predisposing factors are gallstones in the biliary system or biliary strictures. Acute cholangitis does not usually occur in the presence of malignancy unless infection has been introduced by ERCP. Rarely, cholangitis can result following surgical or endoscopic sphincterotomy. Bacterial pathogens that are usually involved include enteric Gram-negative rods, anaerobes, *Bacteroides fragilis*, and, less often, *Enterococcus faecalis*.

PRESENTATION

The classic presentation is of right upper quadrant pain, fevers with rigours, and jaundice (Charcot's triad). However, localizing signs may be absent, particularly in elderly patients who may present with low-grade fever and malaise. Abdominal examination may be unrewarding apart from some mild right upper quadrant tenderness.

INVESTIGATIONS

Full blood count reveals a polymorphonuclear leucocytosis with a high erythrocyte sedimentation rate (ESR) and C-reactive protein (CRP) level. Biochemistry is characterized by a high alkaline phosphatase level, and

Notes

while the concentration of transaminases may be markedly raised, the level is not usually greater than 1000 IU per litre. Jaundice is variable depending on the degree of bile duct obstruction. Blood cultures are frequently positive, usually for coliform organisms.

MANAGEMENT

Treatment should be commenced with broad-spectrum antibiotics such as intravenous (amoxy)ampicillin 2 g 6 hourly or ciprofloxacin 750 mg twice daily intravenously, gentamicin 5–7 $mg\,kg^{-1}day^{-1}$ once daily, and metronidazole 500 mg 8–12 hourly to cover anaerobic organisms. In some patients, despite systemic antibiotics, suppurative cholangitis can progress to bacteremic shock. In such cases, urgent decompression of the biliary tree should be performed, usually via ERCP, although the percutaneous transhepatic route can be employed when the ampulla is inaccessible. Surgical morbidity in elderly frail patients is high and abdominal surgery should be avoided if possible.

Management of common duct stones is covered in *Section 1.5.33.*

Pancreatic Disease

1.6.1

Acute Pancreatitis

EPIDEMIOLOGY AND PATHOGENESIS

The causes of acute pancreatitis are listed in *Table 47*. The effect of the primary insult is to trigger a sequence of events resulting in release of activated pancreatic enzymes from the zymogen granules in the acinar cells. These overcome local pancreatic protease inhibitors and autodigestion of the pancreas occurs. This further damages cell membranes leading to proteolysis, oedema, vascular damage, and necrosis. Spasm or thrombosis of local blood vessels may be additional factors.

Gallstones can induce acute pancreatitis by causing temporary obstruction of the pancreatic duct, producing increased ductal pressure with oedema and leakage of enzymes into the circulation. Retrograde flow of bile or

Table 47 Causes of acute pancreatitis

Gallstones
Alcohol
Posttraumatic (e.g. blunt abdominal trauma)
Viral infections (e.g. mumps)
Drugs (e.g. corticosteroids, diuretics, azathioprine)
Iatrogenic (e.g. post-ERCP)
Ischaemia
Pancreatic tumours
Hyperparathyroidism
Hyperlipidemia
Hereditary
Idiopathic

Notes

bacteria along the pancreatic duct may play a role, although evidence is wanting.

PRESENTATION

Most patients with acute pancreatitis have epigastric or upper abdominal pain and in half it radiates into the back. The severity varies from mild discomfort to excruciating pain, accompanied by nausea and vomiting. Functional bowel obstruction, initially confined to the upper jejunum and transverse colon, is often present. Physical examination may reveal signs of peritonism. Low-grade pyrexia is frequently present with a variable degree of shock. In elderly patients mental confusion is common and signs of respiratory distress, pleural effusions, ascites, and ileus may occur.

INVESTIGATIONS

Acute pancreatitis should be considered in any patient presenting with upper abdominal or lower chest pain. The diagnostic test is estimation of serum amylase, which is usually increased to levels at least five times the upper limit of normal. Raised serum amylase levels are also found in other upper abdominal emergencies such as perforated duodenal ulcer. Estimation of amylase in the peritoneal fluid obtained after peritoneal aspiration and lavage is useful in difficult cases. Ultrasonography or computed tomography may show a swollen pancreas and, performed serially, may provide useful information. They may also identify gallstones and hence determine subsequent management.

Notes

It is important to exclude other conditions such as perforated peptic ulcer, biliary colic, acute cholecystitis, and mesenteric infarction which may mimic acute pancreatitis. A diagnosis of acute pancreatitis should also be considered in patients admitted with hypothermia or diabetic coma.

The index proposed by Ranson and co-workers is useful in evaluating the course and prognosis of acute pancreatitis (see *Table 48*). The scheme uses age and ten laboratory parameters determined at the beginning of treatment or 48 hours after the diagnosis. A severe course is assumed if more than three prognostic factors are present.

Table 48 Criteria for the prediction of severe acute pancreatitis (if more than three criteria are positive the attack is predicted to be severe)

Initial/early findings	
Age	> 55 years
Serum glucose	> 10 mmol l^{-1}
White cell count	> 16 000 per µl
Lactate dehydrogenase	> 600 IU l^{-1}
Aspartate aminotransferase	> 100 IU l^{-1}
Subsequent findings (24–48 hours after disease onset)	
Decrease in hematocrit	>10%
Serum calcium	< 2.0 mmol l^{-1}
Base deficit	> 4.0 mmol l^{-1}
Arterial partial pressure of oxygen	< 7.5 kPA
Blood urea	> 16 mmol l^{-1}
Fluid deficit	> 6 liters

Notes

MANAGEMENT

The treatment is supportive: pain is treated with analgesia such as pethidine; morphine is best avoided as it causes spasm of the sphincter of Oddi and an increase amylase levels; nasogastric suction for vomiting; fluid and electrolytes are administered intravenously. Parenteral nutrition should be considered in severely malnourished patients. In patients with severe pancreatitis multiorgan failure may occur requiring intensive care, ventilation, and dialysis. Treatment with protein inhibitors, such as aprotinin have not been shown to be of benefit in controlled trials, and the use of therapeutic peritoneal lavage remains controversial.

Pseudocysts associated with persistent hyperamylasemia usually require treatment only if they persist beyond 6 weeks. Persistent symptomatic collections can be aspirated under ultrasonographic control or removed surgically. There is a risk of haemorrhage into large pseudocysts.

Pancreatic abscess is an unusual complication arising from secondary bacterial infection of a peripancreatic collection, usually about 10–16 days after the onset of symptoms. Persistent swinging pyrexia, neutrophilia, and a palpable mass raise this possibility and, if patients are deteriorating, surgical intervention may be required, together with broad-spectrum parenteral antibiotics.

Notes

1.6.2

Chronic Pancreatitis

EPIDEMIOLOGY AND PATHOGENESIS

The causes of chronic pancreatitis are shown in *Table 49*. In the developed world alcohol is the cause in over 90% of patients. The mechanism of action is unclear; alcohol might increase bile and duodenal juice reflux into the pancreatic duct or may stimulate excess protein production in pancreatic juice causing plugging of the acini, ductular dilatation, and acinar atrophy.

Chronic inflammation causes progressive exocrine atrophy and fibrous replacement. The main pancreatic duct becomes dilated, tortuous, and strictured. Intraluminal calcification of the protein plugs may occur leading to stone formation. The pancreatic islets are at first preserved but later may become atrophied, due to local ischaemia. The destruction of the exocrine and ductular tissue of the pancreas leads to a progressive fall in bicarbonate and enzyme secretion. However, the pancreas has a large reserve capacity and malabsorption becomes manifest only when more than 90% of the normal pancreatic enzymatic output is lost.

Table 49 Common causes of chronic pancreatitis

Alcohol
Hereditary
Protein energy malnutrition
Congenital anatomic abnormalities
Idiopathic

Notes

PRESENTATION

Upper abdominal pain radiating to the back and worsened by alcohol or food is the main symptom of chronic pancreatitis. There is often severe weight loss due to anorexia. Some patients present with malabsorption without abdominal pain. Other features include diabetes mellitus in 30% with long-standing disease, jaundice due to bile duct obstruction, and portal hypertension due to thrombosis of the splenic and portal venous system.

INVESTIGATIONS

Ultrasonography is the first investigation, although pancreatic calcification may be seen on plain abdominal radiography in a minority of cases. ERCP is usually performed to confirm the diagnosis and to delineate the anatomy of the pancreatic duct. Pancreatic calculi may also be seen. The serum amylase level may not be raised even during attacks of severe acute pain.

It can be difficult, even after imaging and laparotomy, to differentiate chronic pancreatitis from carcinoma of the pancreas. Pseudocysts may require aspiration by either ultrasonography or removal by surgery. Small cysts are frequently seen on ultrasonography. When the pancreatic duct is severely disrupted pancreatic ascites can occur, and is diagnosed by a high amylase content in the fluid.

MANAGEMENT

Management requires pain relief and replacement of exocrine and endocrine insufficiency. All patients, irrespec-

Notes

tive of the etiology, should be advised to stop drinking alcohol. Oral analgesics are often necessary and some patients may require opiates to control the pain. *Pancreatic enzyme supplements* (see 2.3.3) may reduce the pain, probably by reducing endogenous pancreatic secretion by a negative feedback mechanism. Coeliac axis nerve blockade has been used, although pain relief is only temporary (6–8 weeks). Surgery should be considered in patients with intractable pain, and anastomosing the main pancreatic duct to the jejunum (Puestow procedure) is sometimes effective. Pancreatic resection may be of benefit in selected patients and surgery is required for pancreatic ascites.

Malabsorption due to exocrine deficiency is treated by pancreatic supplements. Fat-soluble vitamin replacement may also be necessary. If steatorrhoea is troublesome a low fat diet is tried, and calorie intake is supplemented by increased carbohydrate and medium-chain triglyceride preparations. If steatorrhea fails to improve with pancreatic supplements then gastric antisecretory drugs (H_2-receptor antagonists or proton pump inhibitors) are added to minimize the degradation of the enzymes by acid. Diabetic management is the same as in type 1 diabetes mellitus, although patients tend to have "brittle diabetes" due to a lack of pancreatic glucagon.

1.6.3

Pancreatic Carcinoma

EPIDEMIOLOGY AND PATHOGENESIS

Carcinoma of the pancreas is the fifth commonest cause of death from cancer in the West. The incidence has

Notes

doubled in England and Wales since 1930; there is a male predominance (1.5:1) and risk increases with age. Known risk factors are cigarette smoking and consumption of alcohol.

Carcinoma of the pancreas, usually adenocarcinoma from duct epithelium, develops in the head, body, or tail of the gland.

PRESENTATION

Pain, weight loss, and jaundice are the cardinal features of pancreatic carcinoma. Pain is present in approximately 60%, is usually epigastric radiating to the back, and is often worse when recumbent and eased by sitting forward. Rapid and progressive weight loss is prominent in over 90% of patients.

Jaundice occurs in about 90% of cases and is the presenting symptom in approximately 20%. Tumors in the pancreatic head are most commonly associated with jaundice but one third of jaundiced patients have tumors of the body and tail causing bile duct obstruction by enlarged lymph nodes in the porta hepatis. Weakness, fatigue, and diarrhoea are common but steatorrhoea occurs in about 25% of cases. Diabetes mellitus may develop and there is an increased incidence of superficial thrombophlebitis and deep vein thrombosis.

INVESTIGATIONS

Ultrasonography is the first-line investigation and may be diagnostic. However, the pancreas is often obscured by bowel gas and computed tomograhpy (CT) can be

Notes

more helpful. CT is also useful in assessing local spread. Endoscopic retrograde cholangiopancreatography (ERCP) confirms the diagnosis and aspiration cytology can be performed. Biopsy or fine-needle aspiration of the pancreatic mass can be performed either at CT or ultrasonography. Angiography is required if pancreatic resection is to be considered. No reliable serum markers exist and amylase levels may be normal.

MANAGEMENT

Resection of the tumour is possible in less than 20% of patients. Jaundice can be relieved by endoscopic or transhepatic stenting. Surgical bypass is used when these techniques are not possible or unavailable. The majority of tumours are unresponsive to available chemotherapy or radiotherapy, although trials are in progress.

Survival following diagnosis is generally less than 6 months. Even in patients considered operable, the 5-year survival rate is only 2%. The prognosis for ampullary tumours is better: 40% are suitable for radical surgery and the survival rate is 60% at 2 years and 30% at 5 years.

SECTION B

Oesophageal and Gastroduodenal Medication	2.1
Small and Large Intestinal Medications	2.2
Hepatobiliary and Pancreatic Medication	2.3
Immunosuppresive Medication	2.4

Oesophageal and Gastroduodenal Medication

2.1

2.1.1

Antacids

PHARMACOLOGY

Antacids are basic compounds that neutralize intragastric acidity. The associated rise in pH is believed to explain the therapeutic effect. There are a multitude of different combinations of agents that make up the category of antacids. Antacids are often of complex chemical constituents including magnesium, calcium, and aluminium salts, as either bicarbonates, carbonates, or hydroxides. Some agents also contain local anaesthetic agents, silicone or alginate. It is thus impossible to be sure that all antacids are equal in therapeutic efficacy although this assumption is generally made.

CLINICAL USE AND INDICATIONS

- Symptom relief of heartburn and postprandial indigestion.
- Peptic ulcer healing.
- Prophylaxis of stress-related erosions or ulcers.
- (Phosphorus depletion, by formation of insoluble complexes with aluminium ions, in patients with chronic renal failure).

DOSAGE

Antacids are generally available at pharmacies "over the counter" and are perceived by patients as symptomatic remedies for upper gastrointestinal discomfort. Thus,

Notes

although antacids are fairly powerful ulcer-healing tools, they are used primarily for as required symptomatic relief in indigestion.

Choice can generally be based on cost and convenience as some preparations are liquid and others are in tablet or gel form.

Heartburn and postprandial indigestion. Antacids are best taken when symptoms occur or are expected. This is usually between meals and at bedtime, three to four times per day. A typical dose of a conventional magnesium–aluminium-containing liquid antacid is 10 ml three to four times per day.

Peptic ulcer healing. High doses of antacids (e.g. 175–250 mmol neutralizing capacity per day – exact doses of preparations producing this vary but generally are not large) given in four divided doses produce duodenal and gastric ulcer healing rates similar to those of other peptic ulcer treatments.

Prophylaxis of stress-related erosions or ulcers. Antacid is given hourly via nasogastric tube to maintain gastric alkalinization (gastric pH > 3.5). Despite this ulceration can still occur.

PROBLEMS AND UNWANTED EFFECTS

Magnesium-containing agents are prone to produce diarrhoea and aluminium products supposedly provoke constipation. The evidence that these unwanted effects are a significant clinical problem is limited.

Massive doses of sodium bicarbonate and calcium (usually from milk) can produce alkalosis leading to the milk alkali syndrome but this is extremely rare these

Notes

days. The sodium content of some antacids is lower than that of others and this can be important in patients on salt-free diets.

In the prophylaxis of stress-related erosions or ulcers there is a risk of gastric bacterial overgrowth and subsequent nosocomial pneumonia.

DRUG INTERACTIONS

Antacids can reduce the absorption of many other drugs by binding in the gastrointestinal tract; by reduction in gastric acidity; and occasionally through faster gastric emptying. It is sensible advice for patients to take other drugs about 2 hours distant from antacid use.

TIPS AND TRICKS

In practice, the cost, taste, and convenience of a preparation should determine choice. Antacids are generally available at pharmacies "over the counter".

2.1.2 Alginates

PHARMACOLOGY

Gaviscon and Algicon are the two major examples in this group. They contain seaweed extract (alginate) which forms a floating coagulum barrier that supposedly protects the oesophageal mucosa from acid and other gastric contents. It is proposed that, with Gaviscon, a raft

Notes

of alginate forms over the pool of liquid in the stomach by trapping of carbon dioxide produced through the reaction of sodium bicarbonate with hydrochloric acid. This raft is then preferentially refluxed into the oesophagus when reflux occurs, lies on the oesophageal mucosa and protects the lining. In addition to alginate, these medications have an antacid component. The neutralizing capacity of liquid Gaviscon, however, is limited.

CLINICAL USE AND INDICATIONS

- Symptom relief of heartburn and postprandial indigestion.

DOSAGE

Gaviscon. 500-mg tablet (2 mmol sodium) or liquid (5 ml contains 3 mmol sodium). A standard dose of one to two tablets or 10–20 ml after meals and at bedtime could give up to 48 mmol sodium daily.

Gaviscon Avanced. Liquid only (5 ml contains 2.3 mmol sodium). The standard dose is 5–10 ml, giving a possible daily sodium intake of 18 mmol.

Algicon. One or two tablets four times daily, chewed after meals and at bedtime. Algicon has negligible sodium.

PROBLEMS AND UNWANTED EFFECTS

There are no apparent unwanted effects although the sodium content of Gaviscon should be considered if very strict sodium restriction is in force.

Notes

2.1

TIPS AND TRICKS

Available at pharmacies "over the counter".

2.1.3

Histamine H_2-receptor Antagonists

PHARMACOLOGY

H_2-receptor antagonists compete with histamine for occupancy of H_2 receptors. These receptors are found primarily in the stomach on the parietal cell and thus the main action is reduction of acid secretion. Histamine is the substance that stimulates the parietal cell activating the cyclic adenosine monophosphate (AMP) system and other intracellular mechanisms that subsequently activate the proton pump. Thus the effects of the H_2-receptor antagonists reflect the background level of histamine with which they must directly compete, and potency or receptor affinity also determines how avidly the receptor antagonist binding lasts. The H_2-receptor antagonists are a remarkably safe group of drugs and it has been calculated that they have been given to almost half the world's population.

Cimetidine

Cimetidine, an imidazole compound, was the first histamine H_2-receptor antagonist released for general use. It is the least potent of the available H_2-receptor

Notes

antagonists and over a 24-hour period it raises mean intragastric pH in patients with duodenal ulcer from about 1.4 to about 1.7. If treatment is continued it appears that the antisecretory effect is somewhat less than after the first few doses. This has been called "tolerance", but may simply be an exaggerated response to the first dose. It probably occurs with all H_2-receptor antagonists and may be of relevance clinically when substantial anti-secretory activity is required long term as in reflux oesophagitis. It is absorbed in the small intestine and undergoes hepatic metabolism and urinary clearance unchanged. Binding of H_2-receptor antagonists on blood vessels, in the central nervous system or elsewhere, is probably of little clinical import. Cimetidine is not effective as a traditional anti-H_1 histamine in allergic reactions. Cimetidine has marginally more problems than the remainder of the H_2-receptor antagonists because of binding of the imidazole ring to hepatic cytochrome P450 enzymes (mainly CYP1A2) with inhibition of oxidative drug metabolism.

Ranitidine

Through chemical differences, ranitidine is more potent than cimetidine and, as it has a furan ring instead of an imidazole ring, it binds less avidly to cytochrome P450 enzymes. Median 24-hour pH rises in patients with duodenal ulcer from 1.4 to 2.4 with 300 mg daily in divided doses. Continued treatment, particularly with higher doses, leads to slightly decreased antisecretory effects, although this "tolerance" is probably of little clinical importance. Metabolism is similar to that of other

Notes

H_2-receptor antagonists with a proportion of drug eliminated unchanged in urine.

Famotidine

Another chemical manipulation makes famotidine the most potent of the available H_2-receptor antagonists. A single dose of 40 mg daily produces similar acid suppression as standard doses of the other drugs in this class. Its activity lasts somewhat longer than the others. Famotidine is a very weak inhibitor of cytochrome P450 enzymes and does not have significant drug interactions.

Nizatidine

Although chemically distinct, the same details apply to nizatidine as to ranitidine. It has no appreciable binding to cytochrome P450 enzymes.

Roxatidine

Roxatidine has approximately twice the potency of ranitidine but is otherwise very similar. It has no appreciable binding to cytochrome P450 enzymes.

CLINICAL USE AND INDICATIONS

- Peptic ulcer healing.
- Prevention of peptic ulcer recurrence.
- Gastrooesophageal reflux with or without mild oesophagitis.
- Nonulcer dyspepsia.
- Prophylaxis of stress-related erosions or ulcers.

Notes

DOSAGE

There is least competition for H_2-receptor antagonists at night when the stomach effectively sleeps and when food is not taken to stimulate secretion. This fact and the finding that high levels of acidity at night typify duodenal ulcer disease has led to single nocturnal dosing with these drugs. Food should be avoided after taking this nocturnal dose as it limits the antisecretory effects. Reflux oesophagitis is logically treated during the day when at least half the reflux occurs.

Cimetidine

A dose of 800 mg at bedtime is as effective in duodenal and gastric ulceration as a similar dose split up during the day. Some 75% of ulcers are expected to heal during 4 weeks' treatment and over 90% after 8 weeks. Half the healing dose long term prevents peptic ulcers from recurring in the majority. However, these two diseases are better treated by *Helicobacter pylori* eradication.

In reflux oesophagitis 400 mg two or three times daily is average therapy but some patients can be given 400 mg four times a day. There is not much evidence to support the use of higher doses. Mild oesophagitis heals in 40–60% of cases over about 8 weeks. Long-term treatment with standard doses of H_2-receptor antagonists are relatively ineffective at preventing recurrence of oesophagitis.

Cimetidine also controls some of the symptoms of nonulcer dyspepsia and is available in low dosage (100 mg) in Europe at pharmacies as an over-the-counter preparation.

Notes

Although cimetidine and the other H_2-receptor antagonists are used in the prevention of stress ulceration, good supportive clinical trial data are lacking except for patients with fulminant hepatic failure. The recommended dosage for cimetidine is 400 mg four times daily by injection (slowly over 2 min).

Ranitidine

Ranitidine, 150 mg twice daily or 300 mg at night, can be used for peptic ulceration, similar to cimetidine. Half the healing dose long term prevents the majority of peptic ulcers recurring. There is some evidence that ranitidine produces marginally better clinical responses than cimetidine.

In reflux oesophagitis 150 mg twice or three times daily is average therapy but some patients need a doubling of this dose to 300 mg for effective control of symptoms. In some countries a 75 mg dose is available at pharmacies without prescription for patients with indigestion and heartburn.

In stress ulceration the recommended dose of 50 mg twice daily by injection may be too low, as with cimetidine. Continuous infusion may be more effective; one regimen is an initial 50 mg intravenous bolus followed by 0.12–0.24 $mg\,kg^{-1}\,h^{-1}$.

Famotidine

Famotidine 20–40 mg daily can be used similarly to cimetidine or ranitidine for the indications above. In some countries a 10 mg dose is available at pharmacies

Notes

without prescription for patients with indigestion and heartburn.

Nizatidine

Nizatidine 150–300 mg daily can be used similarly to cimetidine or ranitidine for the indications above.

Roxatidine

Roxatidine 150–300 mg daily can be used similarly to cimetidine or ranitidine for the indications above.

PROBLEMS AND UNWANTED EFFECTS

Cimetidine. Gynecomastia has been reported, although the mechanism is not entirely clear. It probably has no relevance to the minor antiandrogen effects that have been demonstrated with cimetidine. This side-effect appears to be dose related. Impotence has also been reported but it is not clear that the frequency exceeds that in an untreated population. Central nervous depression leading to a muzzy feeling or drowsiness is probably also a genuine side-effect which rarely interferes with clinical use.

Ranitidine. Few problems arise from ranitidine use. Gynecomastia has been reported although the explanation is unclear. Idiosyncratic hepatitis and renal disease are rarely reported.

Famotidine. Idiosyncratic chest pain, hepatitis, and renal disease are rarely reported.

Nizatidine and roxatidine. There is less experience with these medications; however, side-effects are probably similar to those of ranitidine.

Notes

Other effects of rashes, blood dyscrasias, headaches, and diarrhoea are shared by the H_2-receptor antagonists. Inhibition of gastric alcohol dehydrogenase has been reported to be a potential problem leading to higher than expected blood alcohol levels. This inhibition has been reported much less with famotidine. It is unlikely that the interactions reported would raise blood alcohol levels above legal limits as the interaction is mostly reported at very low alcohol doses. In everyday life it is unlikely that this genuine pharmacologic action is of importance, although in litigious practice a warning would not be unreasonable.

DRUG INTERACTIONS

Inhibition of cytochrome P450 enzymes by cimetidine leads to a reduction in the metabolism of many drugs. This is potentially clinically important with only a few medications where side-effects of a drug are concentration related. Thus cimetidine increases the activity of warfarin, and raises the blood levels of phenytoin and theophyllines with potential adverse effects. Ranitidine has fewer metabolic drug interactions than cimetidine and those that do occur are of little clinical importance.

TIPS AND TRICK

In most countries generic cimetidine is the cheapest available H_2-receptor antagonist. There are relatively few clinical circumstances determined by drug interactions that prevent it from being the first-line H_2-receptor antagonist.

Notes

2.1.4

Proton Pump Inhibitors

PHARMACOLOGY

Omeprazole

Omeprazole is a proton pump inhibitor, acting by disabling the hydrogen–potassium ATPase (H^+/K^+ATPase) on the parietal cell secretory membrane. This prevents the exchange of potassium for hydrogen ions and suppresses most acid secretion. The physicochemical features of omeprazole, a substituted benzimidazole, mean that it is attracted to acidic spaces – hence its concentration after absorption in the parietal cell. It is activated by acid and activated drug is unavailable for absorption so the inactive compound is absorbed and concentrated in the acidic environment of the parietal cell where it is activated. The binding to the H^+/K^+ATPase is effectively irreversible by sulphide bonds to the sulphenamide derivative, with new pump formation leading to a return of normal acid secretion. Its antisecretory activity thus builds up over a few days and disappears gradually over 4 days after the drug is stopped. The effect of omeprazole is a potent suppression of acid secretion raising pH from a mean 24-hour pH of 1.4 in patients with duodenal ulcer to around 5.0 depending on dose. Achlorhydria (a consistent pH of about 7.0 or higher) is not achieved as it is presumably impossible to inhibit all parietal cell pumps at the same time.

Omeprazole has some effect against *Helicobacter pylori*, the mechanism of which is unclear. However, the

Notes

organism contains a H^+/K^+ATPase of its own which may be somehow involved leading to inhibition of the bacterium's urease. Further studies will be required here. An alternative explanation is that omeprazole improves the activity of antibiotics by providing a more satisfactory physicochemical environment for antibiotic action, or increases the effective concentration intragastrically by decreasing gastric secretion. Raising the pH may also improve the action of secreted immunoglobulin thus enhancing host immunity.

The plasma half-life of omeprazole is less than 1 hour and active metabolites are not found in any quantity in the circulation. The biologic half-life vastly exceeds the plasma half-life because of active trapping in the parietal cell. Renal excretion of unchanged drug is a minor part of the clearance mechanism, which is mainly through hepatic metabolism.

Gastrin levels rise during omeprazole use in a compensatory attempt to stimulate acid secretion. This fact has provoked a fear that omeprazole could cause carcinoid tumours in humans after prolonged use. Such tumours of enterochromaffin cell-like origin are relatively frequent in rats and occur with any drug that produces adequate and prolonged hypergastrinemia. They are also occasionally found in humans with hypergastrinemia secondary to pernicious anaemia or, more rarely, gastrin-secreting tumours (Zollinger–Ellison syndrome, see *1.4.17 Secretory Diarrhoea*). When found in humans these tumours run a slow indolent course without metastasis, and spontaneous regression has been reported. The level of hypergastrinemia produced during long-term omeprazole use is an order of magnitude lower than that in

Notes

pernicious anaemia so it seems unlikely that such problems would occur. However, in some patients, particularly when atrophy develops, higher levels of gastrin are found and enterochromaffin cell-like hyperplasia must be considered a remote possibility.

Lansoprazole

Lansoprazole was the second proton pump inhibitor to become available in most countries. It resembles omeprazole and behaves similarly. It binds to the three transmembrane domains of the ATPase, compared with only two with omeprazole. For this reason, or some other, it appears slightly more potent as an antisecretory agent, although this is of doubtful clinical importance. Its pharmacologic mode of action is subject to the same physicochemical constraints as omeprazole with eventual binding through the sulphenamide derivative. It is also acid labile and is presented in the same enteric-coated form as omeprazole. There are fewer data concerning the long-term effects of lansoprazole but one would not expect them to differ from those of omeprazole. It produces a rise in gastrin levels as does omeprazole – simply a feature of potent acid suppression. It is more potent against *H. pylori in vitro*, but there is insufficient evidence to show that this is demonstrable clinically.

Pantoprazole

This is another proton pump inhibitor with similar properties to omeprazole and lansoprazole. There are no significant pharmacologic virtues of one over another.

Notes

CLINICAL USE AND INDICATIONS

- Gastrooesophageal reflux symptoms.
- Mild to severe reflux oesophagitis.
- Reflux-related cough.
- Peptic ulcer healing.
- *H. pylori* eradication in combination with other medication.
- Prevention of peptic ulcer recurrence.
- Prevention of nonsteroidal anti-inflammatory drug (NSAID)-related ulceration.
- Zollinger–Ellison syndrome.
- Prophylaxis of stress-related erosions or ulcers.
- (Emergency anaesthesia).

DOSAGE

Omeprazole

In the treatment of reflux oesophagitis 20 mg omeprazole daily for 4 weeks is initially required. In some patients, especially those with more severe reflux symptoms or oesophagitis, 40 mg (20 mg twice daily) is often needed. For mild reflux disease 10 mg daily may be adequate. Symptomatic response is probably the best means of assessment. Therapy is usually required long term or indefinitely if a reflux-related oesophageal stricture has been present.

For reflux-related cough a dose of 20 mg twice daily for 2–4 weeks is initially recommended with the dose subsequently being tailored to the patient's needs.

In peptic ulcer healing 20 mg is sufficient in most patients, although a few require a higher dose, and a

Notes

double dose generally suffices. Treatment is for 2–4 weeks in duodenal ulcer and 4–8 weeks in gastric ulcer. Omeprazole 20 mg b.i.d. is frequently also a component of *H. pylori* eradication therapy (see *2.1.8 Anti-*Helicobacter pylori *Treatment*) in the treatment of peptic ulcer and the prevention of recurrence.

Omeprazole 20 mg daily is more effective than misoprostol in the prevention or healing of either gastric or duodenal ulceration in the presence of ongoing NSAID use.

In Zollinger–Ellison syndrome dosage requirements are titrated according to basal acid secretion measured just before dosing. Measurement of basal acidity should allow for the fact that it may take 4–5 days to reach pharmacodynamic steady state. An average daily dose would be 60 mg in Zollinger–Ellison syndrome.

Intravenous omeprazole is available in some countries and is used when medication cannot be taken orally. The standard dose is 40 mg once daily by intravenous infusion over 20–30 min.

Lansoprazole

The standard recommended dose is 30 mg daily irrespective of disease. This dose lies towards the top of the dose–response curve and therefore additional increments are not associated with much further antisecretory activity. One may postulate that higher doses might be required in Zollinger–Ellison syndrome or to treat *H. pylori* infection, but the majority of patients with ulcers and reflux would be expected to respond to 30 mg daily used for 2–4 weeks (duodenal ulcer), 4–8 weeks (gastric

Notes

ulcer and reflux oesophagitis). Long-term use of 15 mg daily is effective for control of gastrooesophageal reflux.

Pantoprazole

Licensed indications generally lag behind clinical use and it is likely that pantoprazole could be used in all indications where other proton pump inhibitors are used. Clinical trials comparing the different agents are few and do not presently demonstrate a clinical advantage for pantoprazole. The dose of 40 mg should be used where omeprazole 20 mg would otherwise be prescribed.

PROBLEMS AND UNWANTED EFFECTS

There are no common dose-related effects of note with proton pump inhibitors. In clinical trials the frequency of gastrointestinal symptoms, headaches, and other minor complaints including diarrhoea are no greater than those seen with placebo or H_2-receptor antagonist recipients. However, there is some evidence of an increased likelihood of enteric bacterial infection (e.g. *Salmonella* and *Campylobacter*) in takers of antisecretory drugs. Unwanted effects secondary to hypergastrinemia have not been reported to date. There is no need to alter dosage in patients with renal or hepatic impairment. Omeprazole is not recommended for use in pregnancy or in children, although it is effective in the latter group. Lansoprazole should not be used in children or during pregnancy because evidence of its safety in these circumstances is lacking.

Notes

DRUG INTERACTIONS

Omeprazole, like other imidazole compounds, binds to some extent to enzymes involved in microsomal oxidation pathways (cytochrome P450) but many different enzyme systems are involved so it is not possible to predict family effects. The drugs with which omeprazole has been shown to interact are warfarin, diazepam, and phenytoin but not theophylline. The extent of clinical interaction with the first three is limited but it is recommended that patients are either monitored closely or omeprazole is withheld. An interaction with alcohol has not been demonstrated so special advice is not necessary.

Lansoprazole also interferes with cytochrome P450 enzyme activity. Fewer interactions have been described than with omeprazole. Lansoprazole induces CYP1A (a P450 enzyme) which can result in a reduction in the bioavailablitiy of theophylline. Lansoprazole, however, does not interact with phenytoin, warfarin, diazepam, or propranolol. A possible interaction of lansoprazole with the combined oral contraceptive pill has been reported and until more information is available appropriate advice should be given.

Pantoprazole has a lower potential for interaction with the cytochrome P450 enzyme system than either omeprazole or lansoprazole because of a lower affinity for P450 enzymes.

TIPS AND TRICKS

For patients with oesophageal stricture omeprazole or lansoprazole capsules can be snapped open and the

Notes

enteric-coated granules swallowed without loss of efficacy. In pyloric stenosis, proton pump inhibitors may be less effective than expected if gastric stasis exposes the drug to acid.

Symptomatic response with proton pump inhibitors is usually rapid and has been used as a diagnostic test for acid-related disorders, particularly reflux. A 5-day course of double or triple dose should provide dramatic (if not complete) relief of symptoms by the end of the course. If it has not, then alternative diagnoses should be considered rather than persisting with continued treatment.

2.1.5 Cisapride

PHARMACOLOGY

Cisapride is a substituted piperidinyl benzamide with some indirect cholinergic effects by enhancing acetylcholine release in the myenteric plexus. It does not bind to dopamine receptors. It undergoes substantial first-pass metabolism so that only 40% of a dose reaches the systemic circulation. It does not cross the blood–brain barrier and little appears in breast milk as it is highly protein bound. Cisapride is metabolized in the liver and severe liver dysfunction increases drug levels, as would portosystemic shunts. Renal disease does not affect metabolism or elimination.

Cisapride increases lower oesophageal sphincter pressure and motility, accelerates gastric emptying (when delayed), and decreases intestinal transit times. All these

Notes

effects are relatively limited in extent and subject to substantial interindividual variation.

CLINICAL USE AND INDICATIONS

- Mild to moderate oesophageal reflux disease.
- Ulcer-negative dyspepsia.
- Gastroparesis (often associated with diabetes).

CONTRAINDICATIONS

- Gastrointestinal mechanical obstruction.
- Should not be used in combination with the oral antifungals, ketoconazole, and itraconazole.
- Should not be given during pregnancy or during lactation because safety data are inadequate.

DOSAGE

Cisapride 10 mg three times daily (or 20 mg b.i.d.) is as effective in mild to moderate oesophageal reflux disease as short-term treatment (as effective as H_2-receptor antagonists) and longer courses helps to prevent relapse in mild cases. It can be used as a single agent but is often beneficial in combination with acid suppression therapy, either with an H_2-receptor antagonist (except cimetidine, because of decreased bioavailability) or with a proton pump inhibitor. Few data, however, are available on prolonged therapy.

Cisapride has been shown to improve global symptom assessment in patients with ulcer-negative dyspepsia. The dose is also 10 mg three times daily (or 20 mg b.i.d.).

Notes

The initial dose of cisapride in gastroparesis is also 10 mg three times a day (or 20 mg b.i.d.). This has been shown to help some patients, but may need to be increased to 60 mg or more daily before maximum benefit is experienced.

PROBLEMS AND UNWANTED EFFECTS

Abdominal cramps and diarrhoea are the side-effects most frequently reported, but they are infrequent and of little clinical import. Occasional unexplained convulsions are reported. The motility stimulating effects are inhibited by drugs with anticholinergic activity.

DRUG INTERACTIONS

A potentially serious interaction through interference of liver microsomal enzymes has been reported in combination with the oral antifungals, ketoconazole and itraconazole, and this interaction may affect the whole class. These drugs should not be used in combination with cisapride. Despite increased intestinal transit, formal studies have not demonstrated other significant drug interactions.

TIPS AND TRICKS

If used for functional symptoms remember to stop anticholinergic antispasmodic agents first.

Notes

2.1.6

Misoprostol

PHARMACOLOGY

Misoprostol is a prostaglandin E_1 analogue and its effects can by and large be predicted. It inhibits acid secretion through an action on parietal cell prostaglandin receptors. Among many other actions it stimulates smooth muscle activity including uterine activity with the potential to cause diarrhoea, abdominal cramps, and abortion. In clinical practice these effects may be minimal but limit its use to males and postmenopausal women. Prostaglandins generally share a property known as cytoprotection whereby they improve mucosal defence, probably through a combination of mechanisms including improved blood flow, increased bicarbonate secretion, and increased mucus secretion.

CLINICAL USE AND INDICATIONS

- Peptic ulcer healing.
- Prevention of NSAID-related ulceration.

DOSAGE

- Should not be used in pregnancy and preferably avoided in women of childbearing age.

DOSAGE

Misoprostol is indicated in the treatment of peptic ulcer disease. In clinical trials doses of 200 μg four times daily

Notes

or 400 μg twice daily for 4–8 weeks have been associated with healing rates that approximate to those achieved with H_2-receptor antagonists. This is at the expense of increased side-effects and there is inadequate evidence to suggest that they prolong remission after treatment. Consequently they tend to be used as second- or third-line ulcer-healing agents. While better tolerated alternatives abound, there is little reason to use misoprostol in these indications.

Misoprostol may have a role in the treatment and prevention of ulcers associated with NSAIDs (see also *2.1.4 Proton Pump Inhibitors*). Misoprostol 400 μg daily prevents most of the development of superficial endoscopic ulceration associated with acute and long-term NSAID use, and in one study 400 μg twice daily was shown to reduce complications leading to hospital admissions. It does not prevent the latter completely and a satisfactory economic and clinical case has yet to be made for routine use in such cases. Misoprostol is probably effective in healing ulcers associated with NSAIDs but data here are limited and misoprostol may not be any more effective than other ulcer-healing drugs. In any event the first manoeuver should be to stop the NSAID whenever possible.

PROBLEMS AND UNWANTED EFFECTS

Diarrhoea is relatively frequent, although it is seldom severe enough to withdraw treatment. Abdominal cramps are also a common problem but are rarely severe. These side-effects are dose related and are less likely if the dosage is split to four times daily rather than twice daily.

Notes

TIPS AND TRICKS

Use the lowest dose possible in divided doses to limit side-effects.

2.1.7

Pirenzepine (Antimuscarinic)

PHARMACOLOGY

Pirenzepine, the only available member of this class, is a pyridobenzodiazepine structurally similar to imipramine. It is a selective antimuscarinic antagonist which allows it to inhibit acid secretion at doses lower than those required for the cardiovascular and other unwanted effects of classic anticholinergics. It penetrates the cerebrospinal fluid poorly, so is free from central effects.

CLINICAL USE AND INDICATIONS

- Peptic ulcer healing.

CONTRAINDICATIONS

- Renal failure.

DOSAGE

Pirenzepine, 50 mg two or three times daily, is associated with gastric and duodenal ulcer healing rates similar to

Notes

those of cimetidine over 4–8 weeks. The higher dose is probably better than the lower one, but is associated with some side-effects. Pirenzepine can be used in combination with other acid suppression therapy, such as a H_2-receptor antagonist.

PROBLEMS AND UNWANTED EFFECTS

Dry mouth is the commonest effect and is dose related. Constipation and blurred vision, while both recognized, are rare.

TIPS AND TRICKS

Unlike classic anticholinergics it is not contraindicated in glaucoma or urinary retention.

2.1.8

Anti-*Helicobacter pylori* Treatment

This section describes combinations of drugs. It should be read in conjunction with Section *1.2.6* on *Helicobacter pylori*, as treatment regimens and philosophy are likely to develop over the next decade and the regimens listed below may become rapidly outmoded.

CLINICAL USE AND INDICATIONS

- Gastric and duodenal ulcer only (see *1.2.4 Gastric Ulcer* and *1.2.5 Duodenal Ulcer*).

Notes

DOSAGE

The treatment regimens listed below are a few of hundreds that have been used. They have been selected using the following criteria. Eradication rates are above 90% in clinical trials (but remember that in practice eradication rates are likely to be lower). The regimens are of reasonable cost (using UK pricing) and side-effects are known. These regimens are not the only alternatives but they are what the authors believe to be the "best buys" in 1997.

One-week regimens

1 Omeprazole 20 mg b.i.d. plus amoxycillin 500 mg t.d.s. plus metronidazole 400 mg t.d.s.
2 Omeprazole 20 mg b.i.d. plus clarithromycin 250 mg b.i.d. plus tinidazole 500 mg b.i.d.
3 Omeprazole 20 mg b.i.d. plus amoxycillin 1 g b.i.d. plus clarithromycin 250 mg b.i.d.

TIPS AND TRICKS

Compliance must be encouraged as taking three drugs for 1 week is beyond the capabilities of most doctors, let alone patients. It may not be necessary to split the omeprazole dose and 20 mg overall may be adequate. Clarithromycin-containing regimens are generally more expensive but are useful in patients allergic to penicillin. It is likely that equivalent doses of lansoprazole and pantoprazole would be interchangeable with omeprazole. Tinidazole is believed to be better tolerated than metronidazole but is otherwise interchangeable.

Notes

Two-week regimens

1 DeNoltab q.d.s. plus oxytetracycline 500 mg q.d.s. plus metronidazole 400 mg t.d.s.
2 Ranitidine 150 mg b.i.d. plus amoxycillin 750 mg t.d.s. plus metronidazole 500 mg t.d.s.

PROBLEMS AND UNWANTED EFFECTS

The side-effects are those of the individual agents. Pseudomembranous colitis (*Clostridium difficile*) has been reported and can be serious. An unpleasant taste is a recognized effect of clarithromycin, and rashes, diarrhoea, nausea, and candidal infection are well known problems of broad-spectrum antibiotic use. Nausea and a significant unpleasant reaction with alcohol are features of metronidazole and, to a lesser extent, of tinidazole use. DeNoltab may produce dark stools and patients should be warned.

Regimens for use in children are not well described but tetracycline should be avoided.

TIPS AND TRICKS

There is some evidence that 1 week of the DeNoltab regimen may be as effective as 2 weeks, although it is using this regimen that compliance was shown to be so important.

OTHER REGIMENS WIDELY QUOTED

Ranitidine bismuth citrate is a new drug which combines the antisecretory effects of ranitidine with the properties

Notes

of bismuth salts. A dose of 400 mg provides the antisecretory activity equivalent to 150 mg ranitidine. In combination with one antibiotic (clarithromycin 500 mg b.i.d.) eradication rates are encouragingly high but cost is also high and the tested regimens involve a 4-week course. For these reasons this combination is not recommended despite the potential advantage afforded by using two drugs only.

Similarly we do not recommend the two dual therapies with omeprazole and amoxycillin or with omeprazole and clarithromycin, which need to be given for 2 weeks. The eradication rates reported are surprisingly variable (unlike most other regimens) and the costs are moderately high. Again the advantages of simplicity do not make up for these shortcomings, in the authors' opinion.

ASSESSMENT OF ERADICATION

It is clear that most doctors do not check that treatment against *H. pylori* has been successful. However, there are some patients in whom it is important to know that treatment has been successful (following gastrointestinal bleeding from peptic ulcer, when a recurrence could be disastrous for the individual). In such cases or in patients symptomatic after treatment there are two methods to assess eradication. One involves endoscopy and biopsy, and the other a noninvasive urea breath test. Circumstances and availability of tests will determine which is used but it is important that such tests are performed at least 1 month after the completion of antibiotics, bismuth, and proton pump inhibitors because these agents may allow false-negative results. It should also be recognized

Notes

that patients with peptic ulcer who have symptoms predominantly due to acid reflux may remain symptomatic even after successful eradication of *H. pylori*.

2.1.9

Colloidal Bismuth (Tripotassium Dicitrato Bismuthate)

PHARMACOLOGY

Colloidal bismuth, sometimes written as CBS (colloidal bismuth subcitrate), is a potassium salt of citrated bismuth. The proper name is tripotassium dicitrato bismuthate (TDB). Its mode of action is poorly understood. The compound precipitates on exposure to low pH and thus coats the base of ulcers, perhaps protecting them from further aggressive damage. Alternatively it has been shown in animal studies to stimulate mucosal prostaglandin production and is known to have a bacteriostatic effect against *Helicobacter pylori*. Little is absorbed but, once absorbed, the drug has a very prolonged clearance, measurable bismuth being detected in the urine for up to 3 months after stopping the drug. It is also believed to remain in the mucosa for some time after cessation of oral use.

CLINICAL USE AND INDICATIONS

- Peptic ulcer healing.
- *H. pylori* eradication (in combination with other medication; see *2.1.8*).

Notes

CONTRAINDICATIONS

- Renal failure.
- Pregnancy.

DOSAGE

Colloidal bismuth is an effective ulcer-healing drug either as the elixir 5 ml three times daily or as swallow tablets 120 mg four times daily or 240 mg twice daily. In trials, healing rates with colloidal bismuth have been shown to approximate those with comparator drugs.

An effect on *H. pylori* is postulated to explain the fact that duodenal ulcer relapse following colloidal bismuth is slower than after H_2-receptor antagonist use. This effect is not permanent and on its own colloidal bismuth does not cure peptic ulcer. Colloidal bismuth is used, however, in combination with antibiotics to eradicate *H. pylori* (see *2.1.8 Anti-*Helicobacter pylori *Treatment*).

PROBLEMS AND UNWANTED EFFECTS

A small amount of bismuth is absorbed and it should be avoided in severe renal failure. Encephalopathy associated with bismuth salts has not been a particular problem with this preparation, presumably because so little is absorbed. Nevertheless colloidal bismuth is not recommended for long-term use. The tongue and feces may be blackened in patients using this drug but serious side-effects are rare.

Notes

TIPS AND TRICKS

Warn the patient of the change in stool colour. Colloidal bismuth must be stopped at least 1 month before performing urea breath tests for detection of *H. pylori*.

2.1.10

Sucralphate

PHARMACOLOGY

This is an aluminium salt of sulphated sucrose. It coagulates to proteins on exposure in acid and hence is believed to form a protective barrier over the ulcer base. A small amount of aluminium is absorbed but toxicity has not been reported. Adsorption of bile salts is another potentially beneficial effect.

CLINICAL USE AND INDICATIONS

- Peptic ulcer healing.
- Bile reflux gastritis.
- Prophylaxis of stress-related erosions or ulcers.

CONTRAINDICATIONS

- Renal failure.

DOSAGE

Sucralphate is licensed for treatment of gastric and duodenal ulcers and is generally as effective as other

Notes

agents. The dose is 1 g four times daily for both conditions. Dosage with 2 g twice daily may be equally effective. Sucralphate has no anti-*Helicobacter* effect on its own and has not generally been included in eradication regimens.

Sucralphate is occasionally used in patients with gastritis due to duodenopyloric reflux of bile, although formal trials have not been reported.

In intensive care units the suspension of sucralphate is sometimes given to prevent the development of stress-related erosions or ulcers in a dose of 1 g 4 hourly to a maximum of 8 g per day.

PROBLEMS AND UNWANTED EFFECTS

Sucralphate is well tolerated and virtually free from significant side-effects. The tablets are large and some patients experience difficulty in swallowing them. Constipation, believed to be a property of the aluminium component, is a recognized unwanted effect but is not a major problem.

2.1.11

Tranexamic Acid

PHARMACOLOGY

Tranexamic acid is an antifibrinolytic agent which works by competitively inhibiting plasminogen activation by fibrin. This results in retardation of fibrinolysis, stabilization of the fibrin structure, and increased collagen

Notes

synthesis and tensile strength within granulation tissue. Tranexamic acid is renally excreted predominantly unmetabolized and the dose should be reduced in renal failure.

CLINICAL USE AND INDICATIONS

- Acute upper gastrointestinal bleeding.
- (Prevention of bleeding after surgery or trauma).
- (Prevention of rebleeding in subarachnoid haemorrhage).
- (Treatment of primary or intrauterine device-induced menorrhagia).
- (Hereditary angioneurotic oedema).

CONTRAINDICATIONS

- Severe renal insufficiency.
- Haematuria.
- High thrombotic risk.
- Disturbances in colour vision.

DOSAGE

In acute upper gastrointestinal bleeding, tranexamic acid has been shown to reduce the need for surgical intervention and rebleeding, if not mortality. It can be given intravenously 500 mg 8 hourly by bolus injection or orally 1 g three times daily.

Anecdotally tranexamic acid also reduces bleeding from gastrointestinal telangiectases which can not be dealt with by physical ablation. It is also worth a try in obscure undiagnosed chronic gastrointestinal bleeding.

Notes

PROBLEMS AND UNWANTED EFFECTS

Inhibition of fibrinolysis is likely to increase the risk from disorders provoked by intravascular thrombosis – stroke and myocardial infarction. It does not appear to increase the incidence of these when used in acute upper gastrointestinal bleeding, but is not recommended in patients known to suffer or have suffered from thrombo-embolic disease. It is advised to monitor vision, and regular eye examinations are required during long-term therapy. Nausea is a reported unwanted effect.

TIPS AND TRICKS

Reduce the dose in renal failure.

Small and Large Intestinal Medications

2.2

2.2.1

Antidiarrhoeals

2.2.1.1

ABSORBANTS (KAOLIN)

There are many over-the-counter antidiarrhoeal preparations. These include kaolin, aluminium salts, and bulk-forming medication (see *2.2.4 Laxatives*). They are not recommended for the treatment of acute diarrhoea. Only kaolin is considered below.

PHARMACOLOGY

Kaolin (light) is a nonabsorbable purified hydrated aluminium silicate. It has absorbent properties, producing a firmer stool while decreasing the number of stools and cramps. There is no reduction in the amount of fluid and electrolytes excreted, and total stool volume may actually increase.

CLINICAL USE AND INDICATIONS

- Chronic diarrhoea where the underlying cause is self-limiting or untreatable by other more specific means.

CONTRAINDICATIONS

- Intestinal obstruction.

Notes

2.2

DOSAGE

The adult dose is 2–4 g orally every 4 hours. Kaolin is not recommended in children. If it is to be used, the following dosages apply: in children aged less than 1 year, 1 g orally every 4 hours; 1–5 years, 2 g orally every 4 hours; 6–12 years, adult dose.

PROBLEMS AND UNWANTED EFFECTS

Constipation may occur.

DRUG INTERACTIONS

Gastrointestinal absorption of other drugs may be reduced (e.g. atropine, digoxin, lincomycin, and promazine).

TIPS AND TRICKS

Oral preparations containing kaolin should be freshly prepared. Vigorous shaking of a mixture should always be undertaken before use.

2.2.1.2 BISMUTH SUBSALICYLATE

Bismuth subsalicylate is used primarily in infective diarrhoea.

PHARMACOLOGY

The mechanism of action of bismuth subsalicylate is uncertain. The salicylate component may act as an anti-

Notes

inflammatory agent. The bismuth has an antibacterial effect.

CLINICAL USE, INDICATIONS, AND DOSAGE

Prevention of traveller's diarrhoea: two tablets chewed well four times a day (with meals and at bedtime).

Vomiting and mild diarrhoea (traveller's diarrhoea): 30 ml or two tablets every 30 min for 5 doses; may be repeated on day 2.

Bismuth is one of the substances used for *Helicobacter pylori* treatment (see *2.1.9 Colloidal Bismuth*).

CONTRAINDICATIONS

- Salicylate sensitivity.

PROBLEMS AND UNWANTED EFFECTS

Bismuth subsalicylate is converted in the gastrointestinal tract to bismuth sulphide, which causes a blackening or darkening of the faeces and tongue.

Overuse should be avoided because of the risk of either bismuth or salicylate toxicity. Long-term use of bismuth salts has been associated with encephalopathy and osteodystrophy.

DRUG INTERACTIONS

There is a reduction in the bioavailability of tetracyclines.

Notes

2.2.1.3

OPIOIDS

Opioids useful in the treatment of diarrhoea are the natural opium alkaloid, codeine (methylmorphine), and the synthetic opioids, diphenoxylate, difenoxin and loperamide. Although morphine is also effective it is not recommended for the treatment of diarrhoea, although in very low dose it is sometimes added to kaolin (kaolin and morphine mixture should contain less than 800 µg of anhydrous morphine).

PHARMACOLOGY

Opioids stimulate water and electrolyte absorption. Their antidiarrhoeal effects are probably due to an antimotility effect. Opioids act at the m (and possibly d) opiate receptors of enteric neurons to inhibit aboral peristaltic activity; there is, however, an increase in intestinal muscle contractions. The inhibition of peristalsis increases intestinal transit time. The tone of the rectal sphincter is also increased. The synthetic opioids have the advantage of substantially reduced central nervous system (CNS) activity compared with natural opium alkaloids.

In therapeutic practice, diphenoxylate (2.5 mg) is combined with a subtherapeutic dose of atropine (0.25 mg). Large doses have unpleasant anticholinergic effects, thereby discouraging drug abuse. In high doses (40–60 mg) diphenoxylate has typical CNS opioid activity including euphoria, and physical dependence can occur with chronic usage.

Notes

Diphenoxylate is metabolized in the liver, with the major metabolite being difenoxin (diphenoxylic acid). Difenoxin is about five times more potent than diphenoxylate as an antidiarrhoeal agent. It is also combined with atropine in commercial preparations.

Loperamide is a synthetic opioid that is more intestinally specific than other opioids. It is more efficacious in the treatment of diarrhoea than diphenoxylate. At therapeutic dosage it is devoid of CNS opioid activity, because of affinity for intestinal opiate receptors and because of high presystemic metabolism. In hepatic disease, however, plasma levels may be raised. Little, however, appears to cross the blood–brain barrier.

CLINICAL USE AND INDICATIONS

- Acute diarrhoea – nonacute colitis, nondysenteric.
- Chronic diarrhoea.

CONTRAINDICATIONS

Opioids should not be used in patients with moderate to severe colitis or dysentery, because they may exacerbate the ulcerative process and precipitate the development of toxic megacolon.

In patients with chronic liver disease opioids increase the risk of encephalopathy (constipation will exacerbate encephalopathy); additionally, such patients have increased cerebral sensitivity to opioids.

Notes

DOSAGE

2.2

Codeine phosphate. 15–60 mg tablets, one three to four times daily, not recommended for children. Liquid 5 mg per 5 ml (usually contains other additives), 20 ml three or four times daily; 4–5 years, 5 ml; 6–9 years 10 ml; 10–15 years 15 ml.

Diphenoxylate hydrochloride/atropine. 2.5 mg/0.25 mg tablet, four initially, followed by two every 6 hours until diarrhoea controlled; 4–8 years, one tablet three times daily; 9–12 years, one tablet four times daily; 13–16 years, two tablets four times daily.

Difenoxin hydrochloride/atropine. 1 mg/0.25 mg tablet, two initially, thereafter one every 3–4 hours as needed.

Loperamide hydrochloride. 2 mg capsules (1 mg per 5 ml liquid). Acute diarrhoea: two capsules (20 ml) initially, followed by one (10 ml) after each loose stool; maximum dosage should not exceed 16 mg daily; 4–8 years, 1 mg four times daily for up to 3 days only; 9–12 years, 2 mg four times daily for up to 5 days. Chronic diarrhoea (adults only): initially 4–8 mg daily in divided doses, adjusted according to response.

PROBLEMS AND UNWANTED EFFECTS

Codeine may cause respiratory depression. Bronchoconstriction has also been observed after large doses. See Contraindications.

Notes

DRUG INTERACTIONS

Codeine, difenoxin, and diphenoxylate potentiate the effects of CNS depressants, such as alcohol, barbiturates, and some tranquilizers.

Concurrent treatment with diphenoxylate and monoamine oxidase inhibitors may precipitate a hypertensive crisis.

No interactions between loperamide and other drugs have been described.

2.2.2 Oral Rehydration Solutions

PHARMACOLOGY

The main constituents of oral rehydration solutions (ORSs) are sodium, potassium, chloride, glucose, bicarbonate, citrate, and lactate. The principle of oral rehydration therapy (ORT) is that sodium–glucose cotransport in the small intestine remains functional in patients with acute infectious diarrhoea. Water absorption occurs passively and is secondary to the active transport of electrolytes.

Preparations are available as powder made up in fresh water before ingestion, or as a ready-made aqueous solution. The World Health Organization ORS preparations contain sodium 90 $\text{mmol}\,\text{l}^{-1}$. Other commercial preparations contain sodium 35–75 $\text{mmol}\,\text{l}^{-1}$. The glucose content ranges between 91 and 200 $\text{mmol}\,\text{l}^{-1}$, and the osmolality is between 249 and 331 $\text{mOsm}\,\text{kg}^{-1}$.

Notes

CLINICAL USE AND INDICATIONS

The main use for ORT is to rehydrate patients with acute diarrhoea. Rehydration of the elderly, of burns victims, intensive care patients and postoperative patients, are other indications.

CONTRAINDICATIONS

If severe dehydration or persistent vomiting does not allow the adequate intake of fluids, then intravenous therapy should be used rather than ORT.

DOSAGE

The amount of ORS to be used can be calculated by estimating the degree of dehydration (*Table 50*). ORS is appropriate if the degree of dehydration is less than 10%. If there is severe dehydration then replacement should be intravenous. The state of hydration should be reassessed after 4–6 hours and, if rehydration is adequate, further administration of ORS should be sufficient to replace ongoing losses (diarrhoea, vomiting, urinary and insensible losses). ORS powders should be reconstituted in clean drinking water. The correct dilution is important.

PROBLEMS AND UNWANTED EFFECTS

Adverse effects of ORT are hyponatremia or hypernatremia, and hypokalemia or hyperkalemia. Hypernatremia is an important risk to neonates and young infants, especially when high sodium ORS (i.e. WHO ORS) is

Notes

Table 50 Dehydration and replacement

Degree of dehydration	Signs	Percentage weight loss	Immediate fluid replacement
Mild	Thirst; mild oliguria; alert	<3	50 ml kg^{-1} body weight orally in 6 hours
Moderate	Marked thirst and oliguria; restless; dry mouth, depressed fontanelle; sunken eyes, reduced skin turgor; tachycardia but normal blood pressure	3–10	100 ml kg^{-1} body weight orally in 6 hours
Severe	Drowsy and limp; rapid feeble pulse and hypotension; increased respiratory rate; sunken fontanelle and marked reduced skin turgor; anuria	>10	100 ml kg^{-1} body weight intravenously in 4–6 hours (if I.V. line cannot be established in a child then 50 ml kg^{-1} body weight intraperitoneally to 1 maximum of 300 ml) *plus* 100 ml kg^{-1} body weight orrally in 6 hours

Notes

used without access to free water. After initial rehydration the WHO ORSs should be used with extra water (at least 2:1 with ORS).

DRUG INTERACTIONS

None has been described.

TIPS AND TRICKS

Vomiting is common in acute diarrhoeal disease and may persist or worsen with ORT. To minimize this the ORS should be given in small amounts at short intervals (5–10 min). If vomiting persists, than intravenous therapy is indicated. Antiemetics should not be given to children.

If proprietary ORS is not available then half a teaspoon of sodium bicarbonate, half a teaspoon of salt, two tablespoons of honey (or four tablespoons of sugar), and a glass of fruit juice made up to 1 litre with pure water (alternatively one part fruit juice with four parts pure water) is a reasonable alternative.

2.2.3
Antispasmodics

Antispasmodics have smooth muscle relaxant properties either by antimuscarinic activity, by a direct or indirect relaxant action on smooth muscle, or by a combination of the above. They may be useful in the relief of pain associated with conditions such as irritable bowel syndrome or diverticular disease. Drugs used in clinical

Notes

practice include the belladonna alkaloid, *hyoscine butylbromide* (scopolamine butylbromide); synthetic antimuscarinics, such as *dicyclomine hydrochloride*, mepenzolate bromide, pipenzolate bromide, *poldine methylsulphate*, and *propantheline bromide*; and other antispasmodics, such as alverine citrate, *mebeverine hydrochloride*, and *peppermint oil*. Those *italicized* are discussed below.

2.2.3.1

DICYCLOMINE HYDROCHLORIDE

PHARMACOLOGY

Dicyclomine hydrochloride is a competitive muscarinic receptor antagonist at gut cholinergic receptors; its activity is much less marked than that of atropine. It probably also has a direct antispasmodic effect on smooth muscle.

CLINICAL USE AND INDICATIONS

- Irritable bowel syndrome.
- Infantile colic.
- (Urinary incontinence due to unstable detrusor muscle).

CONTRAINDICATIONS

- Glaucoma; paralytic ileus.
- Caution needed in patients with gastrooesophageal reflux or prostatic hypertrophy.

Notes

- Dicyclomine should not be used in young infants because of reports of acute respiratory and neurologic disturbances in children up to 10 weeks of age.

DOSAGE

10 mg tablet, 20 mg tablet, or 10 mg per 5 ml syrup. Parenteral preparation (10 $mg\,ml^{-1}$) for intramuscular use only, when oral dosage not tolerated.

Irritable bowel. 10–20 mg three to four times daily. Can be increased until minor atropine-like side-effects occur (approximately 70% of subjects at a dose of 160 mg per day).

Infantile colic. 6–24 months, 5–10 mg up to four times daily, 15 min before feeds; 2–12 years, 10 mg three times daily.

PROBLEMS AND UNWANTED EFFECTS

Because dicyclomine has anticholinergic properties it can aggravate glaucoma or gastrooesophageal reflux symptoms, and cause urinary retention, especially if there is prostatic enlargement.

An effective dose in irritable bowel syndrome is often associated with anticholinergic side-effects. Minor side-effects include dryness of the mouth, thirst, inhibition of sweating, and tachycardia. More marked side-effects include blurring of near vision (impaired accommodation), difficulty with micturition, headache, skin flushing, and CNS disturbance (restlessness, fatigue, excitement, ataxia, hallucinations, delirium, and coma).

Notes

2.2.3.2

PROPANTHELINE BROMIDE AND POLDINE METHYLSULPHATE

PHARMACOLOGY

The pharmacology of these antimuscarinics and their agents is similar to that of *dicyclomine*. Propantheline and poldine are quaternary ammonium compounds which, while less lipid soluble, are less likely to provoke central effects but still have peripheral antimuscarinic activity with expected unwanted effects. Some patients derive benefit from their use.

DOSAGE

Oral: One to two tablets three or four times daily (maximum of eight tablets per day).

PROBLEMS AND UNWANTED EFFECTS

See atropine-like side-effects under Dicyclomine hydrochloride.

DRUG INTERACTIONS

May interact with digoxin, narcotic analgesics, type I antiarrhythmics, antihistamines, phenothiazines, tricyclic antidepressants, psychoactive drugs, and corticosteroids.

Notes

2.2

2.2.3.3

HYOSCINE BUTYLBROMIDE (SCOPOLAMINE BUTYLBROMIDE)

PHARMACOLOGY

Hyoscine butylbromide is a belladonna alkaloid which is a competitive muscarinic receptor antagonist. Its most pronounced effect is relaxation of intestinal smooth muscle. It does not cross the blood–brain barrier and hence has no central effects. The peripheral anticholinergic effects of hyoscine butylbromide are less marked and of shorter duration than those of atropine.

CLINICAL USE AND INDICATIONS

- Irritable bowel syndrome.
- Biliary colic.
- As an aid to radiologic or endoscopic investigation.
- (During anaesthesia).

CONTRAINDICATIONS

- Glaucoma; paralytic ileus; prostatic hypertrophy.
- Avoid in acute porphyria.

DOSAGE

10 mg tablet, 20 $mg\,ml^{-1}$ injection.

Irritable bowel. 10 mg three times daily. Can be increased until minor atropine-like side-effects occur. Intravenous infusion of 5 mg per hour may be useful for acute relief of pain associated with intestinal spasm.

Notes

Biliary colic. Intravenous administration, either as a stat 20–40 mg dose or as an infusion (5 mg per hour) may relieve biliary colic. It will reduce the rise in bile duct pressure caused by morphine.

Radiologic or endoscopic investigation. Intravenous administration in 20–40 mg increments produces significant gastrointestinal relaxation.

PROBLEMS AND UNWANTED EFFECTS

See atropine-like side-effects under Dicyclomine hydrochloride.

DRUG INTERACTIONS

Hyoscine butylbromide may significantly delay the intestinal transit of medication. This includes a delay in oesophageal transit.

2.2.3.4 MEBEVERINE HYDROCHLORIDE

PHARMACOLOGY

Mebeverine hydrochloride is a competitive muscarinic receptor antagonist at gut cholinergic receptors; it is 10 to 20 times less potent than atropine. It also has an indirect antispasmodic effect on smooth muscle.

CLINICAL USE AND INDICATIONS

- Irritable bowel syndrome.
- Gastrointestinal spasm.

Notes

2.2

CONTRAINDICATIONS

- Paralytic ileus.
- Avoid in acute porphyria.

DOSAGE

135 mg tablet, 50 mg per 5 ml liquid.

Adults and children over 10 years: one tablet (15 ml) three times daily 20 min before meals.

PROBLEMS AND UNWANTED EFFECTS

Anticholinergic side-effects are theoretically a potential problem but in clinical use do not seem to occur. Avoid if gastrooesophageal reflux as lower oesophageal sphincter tone is decreased.

2.2.3.5

PEPPERMINT OIL

PHARMACOLOGY

Menthol, the major constituent of peppermint oil, has properties similar to the calcium channel antagonists, and inhibits the influx of Ca^{2+} ions in smooth muscle.

CLINICAL USE AND INDICATIONS

- Irritable bowel syndrome.
- (To reduce colonic spasm during endoscopy).

Notes

CONTRAINDICATIONS

- Ulcerative colitis.
- Paralytic ileus.
- Sensitivity to menthol.

DOSAGE

0.2 ml capsules. One or two capsules, swallowed whole with water, three times daily 20 min before meals.

PROBLEMS AND UNWANTED EFFECTS

Peppermint oil occasionally causes heartburn. Rarely allergic reactions including rash, headache, bradycardia, muscle tremour, or ataxia may occur.

2.2.4 Laxatives

2.2.4.1 BULK-FORMING LAXATIVES

The most satisfactory treatment for simple constipation is a diet rich in fiber. Dietary fiber can be supplemented by *bulk-forming laxatives* which include both natural and synthetic polysaccharides, celluloses, and gums, including bran, ispaghula/psyllium derivates, methylcellulose, and sterculia; and the synthetic resin polycarbophil. Onset of effect is 12–72 hours.

Notes

2.2

PHARMACOLOGY

Bran contains more than 40% dietary fiber. Dietary fiber is defined as plant polysaccharides and lignin which are resistant to hydrolysis by human digestive enzymes. Dietary fiber is partially or completely fermented by colonic bacteria, leading to increased faecal bulk which reduces colonic transit time. Fermentation increases bacterial bulk. Some of the short-chain fatty acids produced by fermentation may also stimulate colonic activity. Non-fermented fiber increases faecal bulk by retaining water. Increased faecal bulk reduces colonic transit time.

Ispaghula is prepared from the epidermal and sub-epidermal layers of seeds of *Plantago ovata*. If only the epidermis is prepared from seed of *P. ovata* or *P. psyllium*, the preparation is referred to as a *psyllium*. Both preparations undergo significant colonic bacterial fermentation.

Sterculia is a gum obtained from *Sterculia urens* and other species of *Sterculia*. It has similar properties to ispaghula. It also has adhesive properties and is used for fitting stomal appliances.

Methylcellulose is prepared from wood pulp or chemical cotton. It acts by increasing stool fluid content.

Polycarbophil is a non-absorbed hydrophilic polyacrylic resin with a high water-binding capacity.

CLINICAL USE AND INDICATIONS

- Constipation.
- To avoid excess straining at stool, for example associated with haemorrhoids, anal fissure, postanorectal surgery, or solitary rectal ulcer.

Notes

- Irritable bowel syndrome.
- Diverticular disease.
- Mild ileostomy- or colostomy-associated diarrhoea (methylcellulose).

CONTRAINDICATIONS

- Dehydration or intestinal obstruction.
- Should be used with caution in bedridden patients.

DOSAGE

Bran. Crude bran can be added to cereals, salads, and baked foods. Pharmaceutical preparations: 4 to 12 tablets or two to three sachets daily in divided doses, before or with each meal.

Ispaghula/psyllium. 2.5–6.4 g one to three times daily in 150–250 ml fruit juice, water, or other liquid.

Sterculia. One or two heaped teaspoonfuls with copious fluids once or twice daily after meals.

Methylcellulose. Initially 500 mg daily, increased by 500 mg until desired effect, and swallowed with plenty of liquid. Usually less than 6 g daily required, in divided doses after meals. Little fluid should be used if being used for ileostomy- or colostomy-associated diarrhoea.

Polycarbophil. 1 g one to four times daily taken with 250 ml water.

PROBLEMS AND UNWANTED EFFECTS

The most common side-effects of fiber supplementation are abdominal pain, distension, bloating, and flatulence,

Notes

and a worsening of constipation if fluid intake is inadequate. Uncommonly, intestinal obstruction (including oesophageal impaction) may occur if there is insufficient admixture of a supplement and fluid before intake. Mild to severe immunoglobulin E-mediated hypersensitivity reactions (rhinitis, asthma, anaphylaxis) have occurred during ispaghula/psyllium preparation for oral intake.

Ispaghula/psyllium contains significant quantities of Na^+ and should be avoided when retention of Na^+ and water may be a problem. Some products may also contain up to 50% dextrose and should be avoided by diabetics.

DRUG INTERACTIONS

Cellulose can bind and reduce the intestinal absorption of many drugs, including digoxin, salicylates, and nitrofurantoin; ispaghula/psyllium may bind warfarin derivatives.

TIPS AND TRICKS

Care should be taken in the elderly or immobile to ensure adequate intake of fluid and food to avoid bolus obstruction.

2.2.4.2 LUBRICANTS

Paraffin oil (mineral oil) is the only recognized member of this category. Onset of effect is 6–8 hours orally, and 2–15 minutes rectally.

Notes

PHARMACOLOGY

Paraffin oil is indigestible and absorbed to only a limited extent. It penetrates and softens the stool and may also interfere with the absorption of water.

CLINICAL USE AND INDICATIONS

- Constipation, especially in children.

CONTRAINDICATIONS

- Avoid use in bedridden patients and those with swallowing disorders.
- Do not use concomitantly with faecal softeners.

DOSAGE

Oral: children 1–5 ml kg^{-1} up to adult dose of 10–30 ml at night. The dosage is adjusted to allow a soft regular bowel action and is then often maintained long term. Rectal: 120 ml.

PROBLEMS AND UNWANTED EFFECTS

Rectal oil leakage causing pruritus and anal irritation will occur if too much is used. Interference with absorption of fat-soluble vitamins A, D, E, and K. Aspiration can cause lipid pneumonitis, and lead to significant pulmonary fibrosis. Reticuloendothelial lipid granulomas can also develop with chronic ingestion, particularly with the concomitant use of faecal softeners, which enhance paraffin oil absorption.

Notes

DRUG INTERACTIONS

Absorption of fat-soluble drugs may be reduced if concomitant administration.

TIPS AND TRICKS

Administration is best separated from meals and other drug intake to avoid interference with absorption (see above)

2.2.4.3 STOOL SOFTENERS

The members of this category are poloxalkol and the salts of docusate. The main one used in the latter group is docusate sodium (dioctyl sodium sulphosuccinate). Onset of effect is 12–72 hours orally, and 2–15 min rectally.

PHARMACOLOGY

Docusates and poloxalkol have minimal laxative effect; their clinical usefulness is as a faecal softener. These agents act as surfactants, lowering the surface tension at the oil–water interface of the stool, allowing penetration of water and fat. They may also inhibit water absorption from the small and large intestine, and stimulate intestinal fluid and electrolyte secretion, partly through alteration of intestinal permeability. Additionally, the histologic appearance of colonic mucosa is altered, similar to that of stimulant laxatives.

Notes

CLINICAL USE AND INDICATIONS

- Constipation.
- To avoid excess straining at stool, for example with haemorrhoids, anal fissure, postanorectal surgery, or solitary rectal ulcer.

CONTRAINDICATIONS

- Should never be used with paraffin oil.

DOSAGE

Docusate. Oral: up to 500 mg daily in divided doses; initial doses large and gradually reduced. Children over 6 months, 12.5–25 mg three times daily (pediatric solution). Rectal: 50–100 mg as a 0.1% solution.

Poloxalkol. Oral: infants less than 6 months, 10 drops; 6–18 months, 15 drops; 18–36 months, 25 drops; three times daily.

PROBLEMS AND UNWANTED EFFECTS

Cramping pains are occasionally reported. There is concern about potential toxicity because docusate sodium is absorbed and excreted in the bile, and has cytotoxic effects on cultured liver cells.

DRUG INTERACTIONS

Concomitant administration increases absorption of some drugs (e.g. paraffin oil and phenophthalein).

Notes

2.2

2.2.4.4
SALINE LAXATIVES

Saline laxatives contain magnesium cations or phosphate anions. Whether used orally or rectally they have a reasonably rapid onset of action. Onset of effect is 30 min to 6 hours orally, and 2–15 min rectally.

PHARMACOLOGY

The mechanism of action of these salts is uncertain. Because they are poorly absorbed, they probably have an osmotic effect, resulting in water retention which stimulates peristalsis. Additionally the effect of magnesium preparations could be mediated partly through the release of cholecystokinin, which results in a net increase in luminal fluid and electrolytes, and increases intestinal motility.

CLINICAL USE AND INDICATIONS

- Chronic constipation.
- Bowel clearance before radiology, endoscopy, and surgery (phosphate salts).

CONTRAINDICATIONS

- Renal impairment (creatinine > 0.2 mmol l^{-1} (or 2 mg dl^{-1})); symptomatic congestive heart failure.
- Sodium phosphate should not be used by pregnant or breastfeeding women.

Notes

DOSAGE

Magnesium citrate. Oral: sachet dissolved in water, 11–25 g daily.

Magnesium hydroxide. Oral: liquid, 15–50 ml daily; tablets, 1.8–4.8 g daily.

Magnesium sulphate. Oral: powder dissolved in fluid, 5–30 g daily.

Sodium phosphate. Oral: liquid, 20 ml with ample water; children 6–9 years, 5 ml; 10 years or more, 10 ml; purgative, adult dose 45 ml, repeated 10–12 hours later. Rectal: one suppository inserted 30 min before evacuation; or enema.

PROBLEMS AND UNWANTED EFFECTS

Some absorption of the component ions of saline laxatives occurs. Thus, they should be used with caution in patients with renal impairment, cardiac failure, ascites, colostomy, pre-existing electrolyte disturbance, or those receiving diuretics. Monitoring may be necessary for hypermagnesaemia, hyperphosphataemia, hypocalcaemia, hypokalaemia, and hypernatraemia. Of note is that the potential toxicity of sodium phosphate may be enhanced in ischaemic colitis.

DRUG INTERACTIONS

Magnesium salts may interfere with the absorption of other drugs when taken concomitantly.

Notes

2.2.4.5

ISOTONIC ELECTROLYTE SOLUTIONS

PHARMACOLOGY

These preparations contain polyethylene glycol (PEG), sodium sulphate, sodium bicarbonate, sodium chloride, and potassium chloride in an isotonic solution. Oral ingestion of large volumes of essentially nonabsorbable fluid produces catharsis and cleansing of the bowel.

CLINICAL USE AND INDICATIONS

- Bowel clearance before radiology, endoscopy, and surgery.
- Used to a limited extent for the treatment of intractable constipation.

CONTRAINDICATIONS

- Gastrointestinal obstruction or perforation; delayed gastric emptying; severe colitis or toxic megacolon.
- Should be used with caution in patients prone to aspiration or gastrooesophageal reflux, and in pregnancy.

DOSAGE

Powder that is reconstituted in water: one sachet in 1 litre. Give 3–4 litres orally over 3–4 hours on the evening (or early morning) before a morning (or afternoon) procedure.

Notes

PROBLEMS AND UNWANTED EFFECTS

May cause nausea and vomiting.

2.2.4.6
HYPEROSMOTIC LAXATIVES

The agents in this class are glycerol (glycerin), lactitol, lactulose, and sorbitol. Onset of effect is 24–48 hours orally, and 15–60 min rectally.

PHARMACOLOGY

Glycerol is absorbed orally but, when given rectally, has an osmotic effect to soften and lubricate the passage of faecal material. It may also stimulate rectal contractions.

Lactulose, lactitol, and sorbitol are nonabsorbable sugars. Lactitol and lactulose are semisynthetic disaccharides; sorbitol is a polyalcohol of sorbose. Other sugars that are contained in small amounts include galactose and lactose (lactulose), and fructose (sorbitol). These laxatives produce an osmotic diarrhoea. Bacterial metabolism of lactulose/lactitol (lactic and acetic acid production) also lowers the faecal pH, which enhances faecal ammonia excretion because of luminal trapping of ammonia as NH_4^+.

CLINICAL USE AND INDICATIONS

- Constipation.
- Hepatic encephalopathy.

Notes

2.2

CONTRAINDICATIONS

- Galactosemia.
- Disaccharidase deficiency.

DOSAGE

Lactulose/lactitol. Constipation: 15 ml orally twice daily, adjusted according to need, up to 200 ml daily; children less than 1 year, 5 ml; 1–6 years, 10 ml, 7–14 years, 15 ml, daily for 3 days then reduce. Enema, 120 ml of 25–30% solution. Hepatic encephalopathy: 30–50 ml three to four times daily, adjust to produce two or three soft stools daily.

Sorbitol. 20 ml three times daily, adjusted according to need.

Glycerol. One suppository moistened with water before use; different sizes for infants, children, and adults. Enema, 5–15 ml of 80% solution.

PROBLEMS AND UNWANTED EFFECTS

Flatulence, cramps, and abdominal discomfort may occur, especially when therapy is initiated. The sweet taste of lactulose may cause nausea. Excessive dosage can cause diarrhoea, and loss of fluid and potassium. Glycerol may cause rectal discomfort and burning, or local hyperemia with minor bleeding.

DRUG INTERACTIONS

Reduced colonic pH may prevent the release of mesalazine from pH-dependent preparations.

Notes

2.2.4.7

STIMULANT LAXATIVES

These are the largest class of laxatives and among the most potent purgative agents. Excessive use can have significant adverse effects. Thus, they should usually be restricted to the short-term relief of exacerbations of constipation. The main groups in this class are the anthraquinones, polyphenolic drugs, castor oil, and dehydrocholic acid. Onset of effect is 6–12 hours orally, and 15–60 min rectally.

PHARMACOLOGY

Anthraquinones are derived from plants and include aloe, casanthranol, cascara, and senna. Other less effective members, which may be contained in combination preparations, are aloin, frangula, and rheum (rhubarb). The only synthetic member, danthron, is no longer available for use in some countries because of concern regarding hepatic and intestinal carcinogenicity with chronic use in mice. The anthraquinones stimulate colonic peristalsis and induce net fluid secretion.

Polyphenolic (diphenylmethane) laxatives are bisacodyl and phenolphthalein. They stimulate small and large intestinal fluid and electrolyte secretion, and colonic peristalsis. Up to 15% of phenolphthalein is absorbed and excreted renally. The urine becomes pink or red if it is sufficiently alkaline. Some of the absorbed phenolphthalein is also excreted in the bile, which may prolong its laxative effect. Prunes contain a derivative of phenolphthalein.

Notes

2.2

Castor oil, which is derived from the castor bean, is hydrolyzed by pancreatic lipase to the active agent, ricinoleic acid. Ricinoleic acid acts in the small intestine by reducing the net absorption of fluid and electrolytes and stimulating intestinal peristalsis. Castor oil is a violent purgative and should not be used in the management of chronic constipation.

Dehydrocholic acid is a bile acid. It produces net colonic fluid and electrolyte secretion, and is a relatively mild cathartic.

CLINICAL USE AND INDICATIONS

- Constipation. To avoid excess straining at stool, for example with haemorrhoids, anal fissure, postanorectal surgery, or after a cerebrovascular event.
- Bowel clearance before radiology, endoscopy, and surgery.
- As an adjunct to antihelminth therapy (senna plus piperazine).

CONTRAINDICATIONS

- Intestinal obstruction.
- Preferably avoided in children.

DOSAGE

Anthraquinones

Aloe. Oral: 80–100 mg daily.
Casanthranol. Oral: 30–120 mg daily.

Notes

Cascara. Oral: various dosages, depending on formulation.
Senna. Oral: various dosages, depending on formulation.

Polyphenolic laxatives

Bisacodyl. Oral: 5 mg enteric-coated tablet, 10–15 mg for adults, 5–10 mg for children (0.3 mg kg^{-1}). Rectal: 10 mg suppository for adults, 5 mg suppository for children; suspension (10 mg per 30 ml), same dose as for suppositories.
Phenolphthalein. Oral: various dosage formulations, usual dose is 30–200 mg for adults, 15–60 mg for children.

Castor oil

Oral: administered when the stomach is empty, adult dose 15–60 ml for a cathartic effect.

Dehydrocholic acid

Oral: adult dose 750 mg to 1.5 g daily in three divided doses.

PROBLEMS AND UNWANTED EFFECTS

The most common side-effects include abdominal cramp, diarrhoea, and electrolyte abnormalities. Suppositories can cause local irritation. Chronic anthraquinone use is associated with dark pigmentation of the colonic mucosa (melanosis coli).

Long-term use of stimulant laxatives is associated with damage to the myenteric plexus with development of an

Notes

inert, dilated aperistaltic colon ("cathartic colon"). Hypokalemia is also a characteristic feature of chronic use. Other abuse-related problems include malabsorption, protein-losing enteropathy, fever, bone pain, tetany, and finger clubbing.

Phenolphthalein may cause hypersensitivity reactions such as skin rashes or eruptions.

TIPS AND TRICKS

To avoid gastric irritation with bisacodyl, tablets should be swallowed without chewing or crushing, and milk or antacid should be avoided within 1 hour of intake.

2.2.5
Sulphasalazine

PHARMACOLOGY

Sulphasalazine (sulphasalazine, salicylazosulphapyridine) consists of a sulphonamide, sulphapyridine, linked by an azo bond (–N=N–) to a salicylate, 5-aminosalicylic acid (5-ASA, mesalazine, mesalamine). Sulphasalazine is poorly water soluble and only about 12% or less of an oral dose is absorbed intact in the small intestine. Of that which is absorbed, less than 5% is further metabolized, about two thirds is excreted in the urine, and the remainder undergoes enterohepatic recirculation. Thus most of the sulphasalazine reaches the caecum and colon where bacterial azoreductase enzymes cleave the drug to release 5-ASA and sulphapyridine. Sulphapyridine is

Notes

almost totally absorbed from the colon and then metabolized by acetylation, hydroxylation, and glucuronidation with 40–70% of sulphapyridine and its metabolites being recoverable in urine. Slow acetylator or hydroxylator status may substantially increase the amount of free sulphapyridine present in serum and excreted in urine. Of the 5-ASA that is released in the colon, at least 25% is absorbed and rapidly eliminated in the urine after acetylation. About 50% of the 5-ASA is recoverable in the feces (30–60% as *N*-acetyl-ASA) and the remainder cannot be accounted for. The colonic azoreduction of sulphasalazine may be reduced when diarrhoea is present or when antibiotics are coprescribed because of reduced azoreduction.

Sulphasalazine probably acts predominantly as a "prodrug" and sulphapyridine as a "carrier" to deliver 5-ASA to the area of disease. This is supported by studies that have shown that rectal 5-ASA is at least as effective as rectal or oral sulphasalazine in remission induction in inflammatory bowel disease; sulphapyridine, however, is ineffective.

5-ASA can be detected in colonic mucosa, but predominantly in its acetylated form. There is considerable ability of colonic mucosa to acetylate 5-ASA which is substantially greater than faecal acetylation, and which probably occurs in the colonic epithelial cell. Most of the mucosal *N*-acetyl-ASA probably derives from mucosal metabolism of 5-ASA as the latter is more readily absorbed by colonic tissue. In addition, *N*-acetyl-ASA appears therapeutically ineffective.

Both sulphasalazine and sulphapyridine cross the placenta to achieve faetal serum concentrations between 50 and 100% of maternal concentration. There is,

Notes

however, negligible transfer of sulphasalazine to breast milk. The concentration of sulphapyridine in milk is about 40% of the serum concentration in the mother. The amount of drug that either the foetus or infant is exposed to, however, is unlikely to be harmful. Although there is the theoretic risk of haemolysis especially in glucose-6-phosphate dehydrogenase (G6PD)-deficient infants.

CLINICAL USE AND INDICATIONS

Sulphasalazine is used in the treatment of mild to moderate ulcerative colitis, as adjunctive therapy in severe disease, and in the prevention of relapses of ulcerative colitis. Similarly it may be useful in Crohn's colitis and ileocolitis, and in some patients with isolated Crohn's ileitis.

CONTRAINDICATIONS

- Salicylate and sulphonamide hypersensitivity.
- Use with caution in acute intermittent porphyria.

DOSAGE

Oral. Acute attack 1 g four times daily until remission, reducing to 1 g b.i.d. for maintenance therapy. For children over 2 years, acute attack 40–60 $mg\,kg^{-1}$ daily; maintenance 20–30 $mg\,kg^{-1}$ daily. Rectal: suppositories, used alone or in conjunction with oral therapy, 0.5–1 g morning and night after bowel movement. As an enema, 3 g at night, retained for at least 1 hour.

Notes

PROBLEMS AND UNWANTED EFFECTS

Side-effects (*Table 51*) are a major limiting factor with the use of sulphasalazine. These may occur in up to one third of patients on maintenance sulphasalazine, and in up to one half of those on higher doses. Most side-effects are relatively minor, but in 10% of cases they are of sufficient severity to require stopping the drug. Many of the toxic reactions can be related to high serum sulphapyridine concentrations and are two to three times more common in patients with the slow acetylator phenotype, which is present in about 70% of patients with inflammatory bowel disease. Because sulphapyridine is renally excreted, the risk of side-effects is increased in severe renal failure.

The most common side-effects are dose dependent and include anorexia, nausea, vomiting, dyspepsia, headaches, and malaise. They occur mainly in the first few weeks of sulphasalazine therapy and can be managed by reintroduction of the drug at a lower dose and with gradual increases.

Table 51 Side-effects of sulphasalazine

Common	Infrequent	Rare
Anorexia, nausea, vomiting	Rash	Agranulocytosis
Dyspepsia	Fever	Pancytopenia
Headache	"Cyanosis"	
Malaise	Neutropenia	Hepatitis
	Haemolgtic anaemia	Neurotoxicity
Reversible male infertility		Nephrotoxicity
		Pancreatitis
Minor haemolysis		Pneumonitis
Impaired folate absorption		Colitis

Notes

Minor allergic reactions such as fever, maculopapular rash, and arthralgia may occur in about 6% of patients. Bluish discolouration of the skin ("cyanosis"), the mechanism of which is uncertain, occurs infrequently. There have been a few reports of more serious dermatologic and systemic reactions such as Stevens–Johnson syndrome and toxic epidermal necrolysis (Lyell's syndrome).

Male infertility also occurs with sulphasalazine and is probably due to the sulphapyridine moiety. Oligospermia and abnormal sperm motility and morphology are present in about three quarters of men taking sulphasalazine. These changes are usually reversible to normal within a few weeks of stopping sulphasalazine, and probably do not occur with other 5-ASA preparations.

There is a broad range of haematological effects associated with sulphasalazine. Minor red cell abnormalities may occur in up to 70% of patients and are dose related. These include contracted red blood cells and small increases in reticulocyte count and mean corpuscular volume, and indicate mild haemolysis. More severe hemolysis with anaemia with or without Heinz bodies is an infrequent occurrence with high doses of sulphasalazine. Sulphasalazine-induced haemolysis may be more severe in patients with G6PD deficiency. Immune-mediated haemolysis with sulphasalazine has also been seen.

Sulphasalazine, but not sulphapyridine or 5-ASA, also impairs the absorption of most dietary folates, which may contribute to the development of any anaemia. Sulphasalazine-associated folate deficiency may rarely be a cause of severe pancytopenia. There are other rare

Notes

severe haematologic effects that are idiosyncratic in type. Agranulocytosis, aplastic anaemia, and bone marrow necrosis have all been seen in association with sulphasalazine. Other rare side-effects include pancreatitis, hepatitis, fibrosing alveolitis and eosinophilic pneumonia, central and peripheral neurotoxicity, proteinuria, crystalluria, haematuria, and nephrotic syndrome. A colitic-type illness, distinct from ulcerative colitis, has also occasionally been seen with sulphasalazine.

DRUG INTERACTIONS

The metabolism of sulphasalazine is markedly reduced when taken with antibiotics, cholestyramine, and possibly ferrous sulphate and folic acid. Sulphasalazine may interfere with the gastrointestinal absorption of digoxin and folic acid.

TIPS AND TRICKS

In some patients with minor side-effects desensitization to sulphasalazine may be considered. The drug is ceased then recommenced at a lower dose with gradual increments. It is currently preferable, however, to try a newer aminosalicylate.

All pregnant women taking sulphasalazine should also be on folic acid supplements.

Many patients notice less gastrointestinal upset with enteric-coated sulphasalazine.

Notes

2.2

2.2.6

Aminosalicylates

PHARMACOLOGY

Oral 5-aminosalicylic acid (5-ASA) is either denatured by gastric acid or extensively absorbed in the small bowel. Thus new delivery forms must present 5-ASA for release in the small intestine and colon by either slow or delayed release or by using an alternative carrier in place of sulphapyridine (*Table 52*).

Table 52 Oral aminosalicylates

	"Carrier" or Formulation	Site of 5-ASA release
Azo bond		
Sulphasalazine	Sulphapyridine	Colon
Olsalazine	5-ASA dimer	Colon
Balsalazide	4-Aminobenzoyl-b-alanine	Colon
Ipsalazide	4-Aminobenzoylglycine	Colon
Polyasa	Sulphanilamidoethylene polymer	Colon
Mesalazine preparations (time and pH-dependent release)		
Asacol	5-ASA coated with Eudragit S	Terminal ileum and colon
Claversal, Mesalazine, Salofalk	5-ASA mixed with buffer and coated with Eudragit L	Ileum and colon
Pentasa	5-ASA microencapsulated in ethylcellulose	Small bowel and colon

Notes

Oral azo compounds

These drugs are modelled on sulphasalazine and rely on azoreduction by colonic bacteria to release 5-ASA. Consequently the availability of 5-ASA may be reduced by diarrhoea or antibiotics.

Olsalazine (disodium azodisalicylic acid), a 5-ASA dimer, releases 2 units of 5-ASA after azoreduction.

Balsalazide is 4-aminobenzoyl-b-alanine linked to a single unit of 5-ASA. The carrier is less toxic than sulphapyridine and is minimally absorbed after colonic azoreduction.

Oral mesalazine (mesalamine) preparations

These are formulations of 5-ASA coated with a polymethacrylate copolymer or a cellulose derivative to enable time- and pH-dependent release. Coat dissolution occurs in the relatively alkaline environment of the small intestine and colon. These preparations do not require a carrier molecule or bacterial azoreduction for the release of 5-ASA. Because of small bowel release of 5-ASA, there is potential for these medications to be effective in Crohn's disease of the small bowel. As regards colonic availability, in inactive disease azo compounds appear to provide more 5-ASA. However, in the presence of accelerated intestinal transit the reverse seems to be the case, with mesalazine preparations providing more 5-ASA.

Asacol consists of 5-ASA in tablets coated with an acrylic-based resin (Eudragit S). This coating disintegrates above pH 7, which occurs in the terminal ileum and colon, and results in almost 90% of the 5-ASA reaching

Notes

the colon. Release of 5-ASA remains consistent in patients with active symptoms and diarrhoea from the colitis.

Claversal (Mesasalazine, Salofalk) is a 5-ASA tablet, with a glycine buffer to aid dispersion, coated with Eudragit L resin. This resin disintegrates at pH 6 with release of 5-ASA in the distal small bowel and colon. The majority of the 5-ASA is released in the colon.

Rowasa I is also an Eudragit L-coated tablet of 5-ASA, but has had very limited study as an oral preparation.

Pentasa comprises microgranules of 5-ASA coated with ethylcellulose which was originally in tablet form but is now encapsulated. This preparation allows release of 5-ASA throughout the gut.

CLINICAL USE AND INDICATIONS

Several of these new preparations appear to be effective in mild to moderate active ulcerative colitis and in maintenance of remission. They may also be effective in Crohn's disease.

CONTRAINDICATIONS

- Salicylate hypersensitivity.
- Therapeutic enteral doses of 5-ASA may be nephrotoxic in humans, and 5-ASA should be used with caution in patients with renal impairment because of its structural similarity to aspirin and phenacetin.

DOSAGE

Olsalazine. Oral: 250 mg capsules. Acute attack 1–3 g daily in divided doses (maximum single dose 1 g) until

Notes

remission. Beginning at the lower dose and increasing over 1 week may reduce the likelihood of watery diarrhoea. Maintenance therapy 500 mg b.i.d.

Mesalazine. Claversal, Salofalk – Oral: 250 or 400 mg tablets. Acute attack six tablets daily in three divided doses until remission. Maintenance therapy three to six tablets daily in divided doses. Rectal: suppositories, 250 or 500 mg (Asacol), used alone or in conjunction with oral therapy, three to six daily in divided doses (maximum of three suppositories of 500 mg), with last dose at night after bowel movement.

Pentasa – Oral: 250 or 500 mg tablets. Acute attack 3–4 g daily in two or three divided doses until remission. Maintenance therapy 1.5 g daily in divided doses. Rectal: enema, 100 ml (1 g) at night, retained for at least 1 hour.

PROBLEMS AND UNWANTED EFFECTS

The side-effects of oral azo compounds and mesalazine preparations are similar, but usually less common, to those encountered with sulphasalazine. For many of the preparations long-term toxicity data are limited. An adverse effect that is more frequent with these preparations is watery diarrhoea. This occurs in 10–15% of patients taking *olsalazine* and may necessitate a dose reduction or drug withdrawal. This problem seems to occur with less frequency with other preparations.

DRUG INTERACTIONS

The availability of 5-ASA from azo compounds may be reduced by antibiotic therapy.

Notes

The pH-dependent release of mesalazine preparations may be inhibited by the bacterial catabolism of lactulose and related compounds because of the generation of organic acids that lower colonic pH.

TIPS AND TRICKS

The watery diarrhoea that can occur with aminosalicylates can frequently be managed by dose reduction.

2.2.7

Enteral Nutritional Solutions

PHARMACOLOGY

Polymeric (nonelemental) formulae provide nitrogen as primarily intact protein (>80%) and carbohydrate as corn starch or maltodextrin. In chemically defined formulae, the nitrogen source is either a protein hydrolysate with oligopeptides and amino acids (semielemental) or a mixture of free amino acids (>80%) (elemental), and carbohydrate is usually a mixture of polysaccharides and oligosaccharides. Fat in enteral formulae is vegetable oil(s), such as corn, soy, or safflower oil. Some formulae may also contain medium-chain triglycerides, which are absorbed more readily than long-chain triglycerides. A guide to nutritionally complete solutions is presented in *Table 53*.

CLINICAL USE AND INDICATIONS

The indications for enteral nutrition are discussed in *1.3.3 Nutritional Support*. Most of the enteral products

Notes

Table 53 Nutritionally complete (clinically non-lactose) adult preparations

Energy content*	Protein content (% energy)	Integrity	Example products	Description
1.0 kcal ml^{-1} (4.2 kJ ml^{-1})	Standard (<20%)	Nonelemental	Ensure, Isocal, Osmolite, Nutrison Standard	Liquid
			Enrich, Jevity, Nutrison Fiber, Ultracal	Liquid with added fiber
		Semielemental	Criticare HN, Pepti-2000, Peptison, Vital, Vivonex	Powder
			Hepatic-Aid II	Powder, essential and nonessential amino acids, low electrolyte
1.5 kcal ml^{-1} (6.3 kJ ml^{-1})	Standard (<20%)	Nonelemental	Ensure Plus, Nutrison Energy Plus	Powder
			Pulmocare	Powder
	High (>20%)	Nonelemental	Traumacal	Powder
2.0 kcal ml^{-1} (8.4 kJ ml^{-1})	Standard (<20%)	Nonelemental	Isocal HCN	Powder
			Nepro	Powder, low electrolyte

* *Values are approximate.*

considered in this section are delivered by nasoenteric tubes (nasogastric, nasoduodenal, nasojejunal), gastrostomy, or jejunostomy.

The most appropriate enteral product for a patient will depend on individual requirements (see *Table 54*).

CONTRAINDICATIONS

The main absolute contraindication to enteral nutrition is mechanical obstruction. Potential contraindications include severe diarrhoea, gastric stasis, enteric fistulae, and intestinal dysmotility. Many of these problems can be overcome, however, by adjusting the mode of delivery or the type of formula.

DOSAGE

Nasogastric and gastrostomy feeds may be intermittent (bolus) offering a more physiologic feed but bolus feeding increases the risk of gastrooesophageal reflux and aspiration. Nasoduodenal and jejunostomy feeds are best given continuously by pump.

Table 54 Enteral product to meet requirement

Requirement	Potentially suitable formulae
Impaired absorption/digestion *or* partial gut rest needed	Elemental or semielemental
Fluid restriction	Energy content 1.5–2.0 kcal ml^{-1}
High energy requirements	Energy content 1.5–2.0 kcal ml^{-1}
High protein requirements	Protein content $>$ 20% of energy
Added fiber	Fiber enriched

Notes

Products with an energy content of 1.0 kcal ml^{-1} can be commenced undiluted in adults. Products with a content of 1.5–2.0 kcal ml^{-1} are best initially diluted to half strength. This reduces the hyperosmolar associated diarrhoea. The strength of solution can be increased in one quarter increments every 24 hours once the final rate has been achieved.

Bolus feeding should be withheld if residual feed exceeds 100 ml. Continuous feeding is started at 40–60 ml per hour. Residual gastric fluid should be checked every 6 hours until feeding is established. If tolerated, the rate of feeding can be increased by increments of 20–25 ml per hour every 4 hours, until the final rate is achieved.

PROBLEMS AND UNWANTED EFFECTS

The most important complications associated with enteral nutrition are shown in *Table 55*. Tube-related problems may lead to aspiration. Diarrhoea is the most common gastrointestinal problem and has been attributed to large volumes, bolus feeds, cold feeds, hyperosmolar solutions, malabsorption (e.g. disaccharidase deficiency), antibiotic alteration of colonic flora with reduced short-chain fatty acid production, and contamination of enteral feeds.

DRUG INTERACTIONS

There is little information available in this area. Some reports have shown that the serum level of drugs such as phenytoin may be reduced by coadministration with enteral solutions. Syrups that contain sorbitol may also

Notes

Table 55 Complications of enteral nutrition

Mechanical, tube related
Improper placement (malposition, endobronchial placement, oesophageal perforation)
Dislodgment or migration
Blockage
Gastrointestinal
Nausea, cramping, gastrooesophageal reflux, vomiting
Diarrhoea, constipation
Infection
Aspiration pneumonia
Infected tract associated with percutaneous endoscopic gastrostomy or jejunostomy
Metabolic
Dehydration
Overhydration
Electrolyte abnormalities
Hyperglycemia

increase the risk of diarrhoea associated with enteral solutions.

TIPS AND TRICKS

Gastric emptying problems may be helped by elevating the head of the bed. Motility stimulants may be helpful. The tube may need to be placed beyond the pylorus. If diarrhoea occurs, the concentration of hyperosmolar feeds should be reduced or an iso-osmolar solution substituted. If malabsorption is suspected with a nonelemental

Notes

solution, an elemental feed can be tried. The addition of 1% pectin (noncellulose fiber) to enteral feeds may reduce antibiotic-associated diarrhoea. Antidiarrhoeals (see *2.2.1 Antidiarrhoeals*) can also be used when other measures have failed.

Hepatobiliary and Pancreatic Medication

2.3.1

Interferon

PHARMACOLOGY

Interferons were among the first cytokines identified and are of three main types: α, β, and γ. The human α-interferons are further subclassified but the subtypes are closely related with conservation of at least half the amino acids in identical positions. Nevertheless they have unique biologic properties. α-Interferons, produced by peripheral blood monocytes, exert effects on viral infections by actions on intracellular viral replication and host immune responses. Upregulation of human leucocyte antigen (HLA) class II molecules on cell surfaces allows viral antigens to be better presented to host T cells. The most commonly used α-interferon is human lymphoblastoid interferon produced by a cell line stimulated by sendaivirus. Alternatives are the recombinant α-interferons, of which there are two currently available.

The time to reach peak concentration following intramuscular injection ranges from 3 to 15 hours and the elimination half-life varies from 3 to 15 hours. Clearance of interferon occurs primarily by renal elimination and/or metabolism.

CLINICAL USE AND INDICATIONS

- Chronic hepatitis B, with or without delta infection.
- Acute and chronic hepatitis C.
- (Treatment of human malignant disease, particularly hairy cell leukemia and multiple myeloma).

Notes

CONTRAINDICATIONS

- Pregnancy.

DOSAGE

2.3

In hepatitis B and D the dosage used is normally 5–10 million units three times a week administered subcutaneously. In hepatitis C a dose of 3–6 million units three times a week subcutaneously has been recommended. The duration of treatment currently varies between 4 months for hepatitis B to 1 year for hepatitis C.

PROBLEMS AND UNWANTED EFFECTS

Toxicity with interferon is common. After the first dose fever up to 40°C, hypertension, tachycardia, severe headache, muscle cramps, nausea, and vomiting often occur. These effects can be reduced by concurrent administration of indomethacin, although this is inappropriate in the majority of patients with chronic liver disease. Concurrent administration of paracetamol is the usual recommendation, and without this, interferon therapy would be intolerable in many. However, tachyphylaxis is marked and patients should be discouraged from stopping therapy at any stage during the course, because reintroduction of interferon will again expose them to the first-dose phenomenon. Neutropenia, maximal at about 10 days, will usual recover spontaneously without any need to reduce the dose of interferon.

Thrombocytopenia is also more apparent at about 10 days and usually remits spontaneously. Within 2–3 weeks

Notes

the main side-effects are severe fatigue, sleep disturbance, poor concentration, mild alopecia, and occasional influenza-like symptoms. A minority of patients develop a severe psychologic disturbance, and depression has been reported necessitating dose reduction or stopping the drug. The presence of autoimmune disease of any type is a contraindication to interferon use, which exacerbates the clinical state. Interferon can be used in children and there is no need to alter the dose in those with renal or hepatic impairment. Some patients, particularly following recombinant interferon therapy, develop interferon antibodies but this is a major problem in only a small minority.

DRUG INTERACTIONS

There are no major drug interactions with interferon.

TIPS AND TRICKS

It is helpful to admit patients to hospital for the first two injections allowing side-effects to be minimized and training under supervision to be given. Most patients can be taught to self-administer interferon. Patients should have antibody tests to exclude the presence of autoimmune liver disease.

2.3.2 Ursodeoxycholic Acid

PHARMACOLOGY

Ursodeoxycholic acid (UDCA) is a naturally occurring bile acid which is present in small amounts in human

Notes

bile. Oral administration of UDCA results in a major alteration in the plasma and circulating bile acid pool. The levels of cholic acid and chenodeoxycholic acid are markedly decreased and ursodeoxycholic acid becomes the major bile acid. Ursodeoxycholic acid, a hydrophilic substance, appears to exert three main effects which may all be beneficial in chronic cholestatic conditions. The first is a choleretic effect increasing bile salt-dependent bile flow. Secondly, it reduces the toxic intracellular effects of increased hydrophobic bile acids which accumulate in cholestasis and, thirdly, it appears to have an immunomodulatory effect. UDCA has been demonstrated to decrease class I expression on hepatocytes following long-term treatment in patients with primary biliary cirrhosis, and in primary sclerosing cholangitis it decreases HLA-DR expression on biliary epithelium.

CLINICAL USE AND INDICATIONS

- Dissolution of cholesterol stones.
- Adult and pediatric chronic cholestatic conditions.

UDCA produces a symptomatic improvement in malaise, pruritus, and well-being, and invariably improves serum biochemistry. However, only in primary biliary cirrhosis has it been shown to prolong time to transplantation or survival.

Notes

DOSAGE

In stone dissolution, UDCA (5 $mg\,kg^{-1}$ daily) is often combined with chenodeoxycholic acid (7.5 $mg\,kg^{-1}$ daily) to reduce side-effects with both agents by using lower doses (see *1.5.31 Gallstones*).

In patients with primary biliary cirrhosis a dose of 10–15 $mg\,kg^{-1}$ per day given as a divided dose two or three times daily, is sufficient. Similar doses are used in adults with other chronic cholestatic conditions. In children, especially those with cystic fibrosis, a higher dose of 20–25 $mg\,kg^{-1}$ daily is needed, probably because of decreased absorption of the bile acid.

PROBLEMS AND UNWANTED EFFECTS

There are no common dose-related side-effects of note, although caution may be necessary when using high doses in patients with inflammatory bowel disease.

DRUG INTERACTIONS

The absorption of UDCA may be inhibited by cholestyramine or colestipol.

TIPS AND TRICKS

It is important to make sure that patients separate taking their UDCA by at least 2 hours from cholestyramine or colestipol, which decrease the absorption of UDCA.

Notes

2.3

2.3.3

Pancreatic Enzyme Replacement

PHARMACOLOGY

Pancreatic enzyme replacement consists of preparations of proteases (trypsin and chymotrypsin), lipase, and amylase which are obtained from animal pancreas, usually the pig. The enzymes when given orally are inactivated by gastric acid secretion and thus new preparations are enteric coated to deliver high concentrations of enzymes to the duodenum. Various methods of delivery are used including microspheres which dissolve releasing the enzymes on either a pH- or a time-related basis. To minimize the number of capsules taken, higher strength versions have now been developed.

CLINICAL USE AND INDICATIONS

- Reduced or absent exocrine pancreatic secretion (as in cystic fibrosis, chronic pancreatitis, following total pancreatectomy, or sometimes with obstructing carcinoma of the head of the pancreas).
- Chronic pancreatitis with normal exocrine function, but with chronic pain. (Approximately half of patients with pain from chronic pancreatitis will respond to some extent to pancreatic enzyme supplementation.)

DOSAGE

Dosage is adjusted according to the fat intake and the number and consistency of stools. In general, one or two

Notes

lower-strength tablets are given initially with each meal, increasing until an adequate response is obtained.

PROBLEMS AND UNWANTED EFFECTS

The most frequent side-effects are upper gastrointestinal, particularly nausea, vomiting, and abdominal discomfort. Hyperuricemia and hyperuricosuria have been associated with very high doses, although these effects are rare. Some patients complain of oral ulceration if the preparations are retained in the mouth, or if large doses are used. Rarely, hypersensitivity reactions may be seen.

There have been a small number of reports of fibrotic strictures of the ascending colon, mainly in boys aged 3–13 years with cystic fibrosis. It has been recommended that patients with this condition should not be treated with high-dose preparations, although the development of strictures has been reported with high- and low-dose preparations. There have been no reports of colonic strictures occurring in patients other than with cystic fibrosis.

TIPS AND TRICKS

The dose may be maximized by giving concurrent acid suppression with a H_2-receptor antagonist or proton pump inhibitor. Some patients find that sprinkling the content of capsules on their food may help, although it should be noted that the enzymes are inactivated by heat. Patients should be reminded to take an extra capsule if they have snacks between meals.

Immunosuppressive Medication

2.4

2.4.1

Corticosteroids

PHARMACOLOGY

Prednisone, prednisolone, hydrocortisone, betamethasone, and dexamethasone are glucocorticosteroids used for their anti-inflammatory effect. Equivalent anti-inflammatory doses are shown in *Table 56*.

Corticosteroids impair interleukin (IL) 1 production by macrophages and as a consequence also suppress IL-2 release from activated T cells. When choosing a corticosteroid for its anti-inflammatory effect, it should be borne in mind that high anti-inflammatory (glucocorticoid) activity is of no advantage unless it is associated with a relatively low mineralocorticoid activity. The mineralocorticoid effects of cortisone and hydrocortisone are too great for them to be used on a long-term basis for inflammatory disease suppression because salt and water retention will be too great. However, they are ideal for adrenal

Table 56 Equivalent anti-inflammatory doses of glucocorticoids

Drug	Equivalent anti-inflammatory dose (mg)
Prednisolone	5
Prednisone	5
Hydrocortisone	20
Cortisone acetate	25
Betamethasone	0.75
Dexamethasone	0.75
Methylprednisolone	4

Notes

replacement therapy when both glucocorticoid and mineralocorticoid activity are required. Prednisolone has predominantly glucocorticoid activity and is the oral corticosteroid of choice for short- and long-term administration. Prednisone has a similar level of activity but is active only after conversion in the liver to prednisolone and is therefore not recommended in patients with chronic liver disease in whom the conversion may be impaired.

CLINICAL USE AND INDICATIONS

- Glucocorticoids are widely used as anti-inflammatories in gastrointestinal and hepatic diseases.
- Liver and small bowel transplantation.
- (Renal transplantation).
- (Connective tissue disease).
- (Respiratory disease).
- (Renal disease).
- (Ocular disease).
- (Blood disorders and malignancy).
- (Glucocorticoid replacement therapy).

DOSAGE

Appropriate doses are discussed in the management of specific disease in *Section A*.

In many cases a dose equivalent to 20–40 mg prednisolone daily is started which is then reduced after 2–4 weeks to a lower dose. In certain conditions, particularly liver diseases, maintenance therapy may be required, usually at the lowest possible dose to maintain the disease in remission.

Notes

In all indications the principles involved in treatment are to use the lowest possible dose for the shortest clinically appropriate period. Thus in inflammatory bowel disease a typical regimen may start with prednisolone 30 mg daily for 2 weeks, reducing at weekly intervals by 5 mg. Many regimens are based on clinical experience rather than evidence that one is better than another. In control of autoimmune chronic active hepatitis, prednisolone is used for many months and in some cases can never be stopped. In such cases the dose used can be between 5 mg and 15 mg daily.

The type, dose, and duration of steroid therapy used in immunosuppression following organ transplantation vary considerably in different transplant units.

PROBLEMS AND UNWANTED EFFECTS

The unwanted effects of glucocorticoids are legion, including diabetes and osteoporosis. High doses are associated with avascular necrosis of the femoral head. Mental disturbances (mania and depression) may occur particularly in patients with a known history of mental disorder. Rarely a serious paranoid state or depression with a risk of suicide may result. Patients commonly complain of difficulty sleeping when taking moderate doses of steroids. Proximal muscle wasting may rarely be a problem and muscle weakness can also occur as a result of hypokalemia. There is a weak association with the complications of ulcer disease. Prolonged use of high doses of corticosteroids may cause Cushing's syndrome, and in children administration of corticosteroids may result in growth retardation.

Notes

Patients who require long-term therapy with corticosteroids have a risk of adrenal atrophy, and rapid withdrawal of corticosteroids can produce acute adrenal insufficiency. Therefore, when long-term treatment is to be reduced, the dose should be reduced gradually over a period of several months.

TIPS AND TRICKS

Soluble prednisolone may be useful in patients with absorptive disorders, and azathioprine (see *2.4.2*) should be borne in mind as a steroid-sparing agent.

2.4.2

Azathioprine and 6-Mercaptopurine

PHARMACOLOGY

Azathioprine and 6-mercaptopurine (6-MP) are cytotoxic immunosuppressants. Their mechanism of action is unclear but they are most useful as steroid-sparing agents, sometimes allowing steroids to be stopped completely. They are myelosuppressive and reasonably close monitoring is required.

Both azathioprine and 6-MP have poor oral bioavailability: about 50% and 16% respectively. Also of note is that azathioprine is 55% 6-MP by molecular weight and that about 88% of azathioprine is converted into 6-MP. Thus, a conversion factor of 2.0 is used in converting from azathioprine to 6-MP.

Notes

After an oral dose azathioprine is rapidly metabolized to 6-MP. 6-MP undergoes extensive metabolism along three competing pathways. A major catabolic pathway is *in vivo* methylation (to 6-methylmercaptopurine), catalyzed by the enzyme thiopurine methyltransferase (TPMT). There are substantial interindividual differences in TPMT activity which are controlled by a common genetic polymorphism. A second catabolic route is oxidation (to 6-thiouric acid), catalyzed by xanthine oxidase. There is probably little interindividual variation of the functional activity of xanthine oxidase. The third route produces several active metabolites, especially 6-thioguanine nucleotides (6-TGNs), catalyzed by the enzyme hypoxanthine phosphoribosyl transferase. These active nucleotide metabolites are cytotoxic and suppress *de novo* purine synthesis.

Many side-effects associated with azathioprine and 6-MP may be related to a very low inherited level of the enzyme TPMT and abnormally high concentrations of the 6-TGNs. Acute severe bone marrow suppression has been associated with very low TPMT activity ($TPMT^L$/$TPMT^L$ genotype). Less severe toxicity, especially leucopenia, may be due to intermediate TPMT activity ($TPMT^L$/$TPMT^H$ genotype). Other haematologic toxicities include macrocytosis, anaemia, thrombocytopenia, and pancytopenia. Cases of late myelosuppression may also represent the heterozygous genotype.

The incidence of haematologic side-effects is similar to the pattern of TPMT enzyme activity in the population: about 11% have intermediate activity ($TPMT^L$/$TPMT^H$ genotype) while 1 in 300 have low or absent TPMT activity ($TPMT^L$/$TPMT^L$ genotype).

Notes

2.4

CLINICAL USE AND INDICATIONS

- Ulcerative colitis and Crohn's disease.
- Autoimmune chronic active hepatitis.
- Liver and small bowel transplantation.
- (Renal transplantation).
- (Immune suppression in autoimmune disease).

CONTRAINDICATIONS

2.4

Pregnancy is a relative contraindication and usage of azathioprine or 6-MP depends on clinical judgment. There is concern, based on anecdotal reports, of chromosome aberrations in patients taking these drugs. There have, however, been a number of reviews of pregnancy in patients who are on azathioprine because of transplantation or inflammatory bowel disease, and no malformation was found in the children.

DOSAGE

Azathioprine is usually used in a dose of 1–2 $mg\,kg^{-1}$ daily, rarely increased to 3 $mg\,kg^{-1}$. 6-MP is usually used in a dose of 1–1.5 $mg\,kg^{-1}$ daily.

For suppression of transplant rejection a loading dose of azathioprine, either by mouth or intravenously up to 5 $mg\,kg^{-1}$ is given, followed by a maintenance dose of between 1 and 4 $mg\,kg^{-1}$ daily.

Appropriate doses are also discussed in the management of specific diseases in *Section A*.

Careful monitoring should be performed throughout the duration of treatment. Full blood count should be

Notes

carried out weekly for the first 8 weeks and more frequently for higher doses or if the patient has hepatic or renal impairment. After 2 months the full blood count should be performed every 3 months. Thrombocytopenia is the first indicant of a significant myelosuppressive effect.

PROBLEMS AND UNWANTED EFFECTS

There are two main types of problem with azathioprine or 6-MP: (1) hypersensitivity reactions; and (2) dose-related toxicity. The hypersensitivity reactions include malaise, fever, myalgia, arthralgia and, rarely, disturbed liver function tests and cholestatic jaundice. Explosive diarrhoea has been reported in patients with inflammatory bowel disease. Arrhythmias and hypertension have also been very rarely reported. The dose-related effects are mainly those of bone marrow suppression (as discussed above), alopecia (which is very uncommon with doses below 2 $mg\,kg^{-1}$), and susceptibility to infection in transplant recipients who may well be receiving other forms of immunosuppression. Upper gastrointestinal side-effects are fairly common, particularly nausea and epigastric pain, and acute pancreatitis does very rarely occur.

DRUG INTERACTIONS

Because allopurinol inhibits the metabolism of 6-MP, dosage of azathioprine or 6-MP should be reduced by 75% when concurrent therapy is given.

Enhanced bone marrow suppression with either azathioprine or 6-MP has been noted with co-trimoxazole.

Notes

TIPS AND TRICKS

In view of the problems with bone marrow suppression patients should be warned to report immediately any evidence of infection, bruising, or bleeding.

2.4.3

Cyclosporin

PHARMACOLOGY

Cyclosporin (cyclosporin A) is a cyclic polypeptide consisting of 11 amino acids derived from a fungus. The predominant mechanism of action is inhibition of transcription of lymphokine genes interfering with interleukin (IL) 2 production. IL-2-producing clones of helper T lymphocytes are the main target of cyclosporin-induced immunosuppression. In addition, inhibition of antigen-presenting cells may be important.

CLINICAL USE AND INDICATIONS

- Liver and small bowel transplantation.
- Inflammatory bowel disease.
- (Renal transplantation).
- (Immune suppression in autoimmune disease).

DOSAGE

Appropriate doses are discussed in the management of specific disease in *Section A*.

Notes

There is some variation in the use of cyclosporin after organ transplantation. Some centers commence cyclosporin beforehand, where as others postpone introduction for 48 hours until renal function has normalized.

Doses usually start at 1mg kg^{-1} per day, increasing to 6 mg kg^{-1} by the sixth day. The dose is titrated to maintain blood levels within a certain range depending on the method used to assess the cyclosporin level.

Cyclosporin is given intravenously for the first 2–3 weeks as absorption is very unpredictable after liver transplantation while bile drainage is externalized or while graft function is abnormal. To achieve comparable blood levels the oral dose of cyclosporin is usually two or three times the intravenous dose.

A new lipid-soluble preparation of cyclosporin (Neoral) has been produced which permits a more stable absorption of cyclosporin and may make it easier to standardize regimens after transplantation. This lipid preparation may minimize the need for intravenous cyclosporin in the peritransplant period. Neoral is given at a starting dose of 6 mg kg^{-1} twice daily.

PROBLEMS AND UNWANTED EFFECTS

Major side-effects are acute and chronic nephrotoxicity and hypertension. The chronic nephrotoxicity is due to renal ischaemia, but has been less of a problem since lower doses have been used. In association with nephrotoxicity there may be renal magnesium wasting, water and salt retention, hyperkalemia, and hyperuricemia. Neurotoxicity has also been described, ranging from seizures to coma, which may necessitate interruption of cyclosporin

Notes

therapy in the early post-transplant period. Headaches, tremour, and paresthesia are common and usually respond to a reduction in the dose of cyclosporin. Cyclosporin is also associated with an increased risk of skin cancer and lymphoproliferative disorders. Oral cyclosporin therapy can cause hirsutism, facial coarsening, and gingival hypertrophy, each of which may be a greater problem in female patients. There is evidence from patients undergoing renal transplant that cyclosporin therapy is associated with intrauterine growth retardation in about half the cases and most units stop cyclosporin therapy for the second and third trimesters.

DRUG INTERACTIONS

Many drugs interact with cyclosporin (and FK506). A pharmacopeia should be checked before commencing any new medication.

The main mechanism of interaction is by competitive metabolism with the cytochrome P450 enzyme system, causing increased levels of cyclosporin (or FK506). This can result in deterioration of renal function, headaches, and tremor. Dose adjustment according to trough levels corrects these side-effects. Induction of hepatic metabolism (e.g. barbiturates, phenytoin, or warfarin) can cause low trough levels of cyclosporin (or FK506), which also require dose adjustment.

Notes

2.4.4

FK506 (Tacrolimus)

PHARMACOLOGY

FK506 (tacrolimus) is a new immunosuppressive agent. It is a macrolide antibiotic derived from the soil fungus *Streptomyces tsukubaenis*. The mode of action is similar to that of cyclosporin; it is active on a cytosolic protein with resulting inhibition of interleukin 2 and T-lymphocyte activation.

FK506 is well absorbed orally and adequate serum levels can be maintained with nasogastric administration. Intravenous usage tends to be avoided because of an associated increased risk of side-effects.

CLINICAL USE AND INDICATIONS

- Liver and small bowel transplantation.
- (Renal transplantation).

FK506 may be used instead of cyclosporin as the principal immunosuppressive agent. In the majority of transplant units FK506 is currently used as supplemental or rescue therapy in patients with acute and chronic rejection.

DOSAGE

FK506 is usually administered in a dose of 0.075 $mg\,kg^{-1}$ twice daily. Blood levels should be maintained at 2–15 $\mu g\,l^{-1}$.

Notes

PROBLEMS AND UNWANTED EFFECTS

The side-effects associated with FK506 are similar to those of cyclosporin, although they are usually less evident. Hyperkalemia tends to be more common than with cyclosporin.

DRUG INTERACTIONS

See cyclosporin (*2.4.3*).

INDEX